COPYRIGHT

Inder Publishing
a division of Inderprint

7C First Avenue, Whangarei
PO Box 4443, Kamo, Whangarei
Ph/fax: 09 430 8002
Email: parkes@inderprint.co.nz

Illustrations by Bill Parkes

2003

ISBN: 0-476-00009-2

INDER PUBLISHING

THE FAIR BEGINNING OF A TIME

BILL PARKES

SHORT WHITE COATS

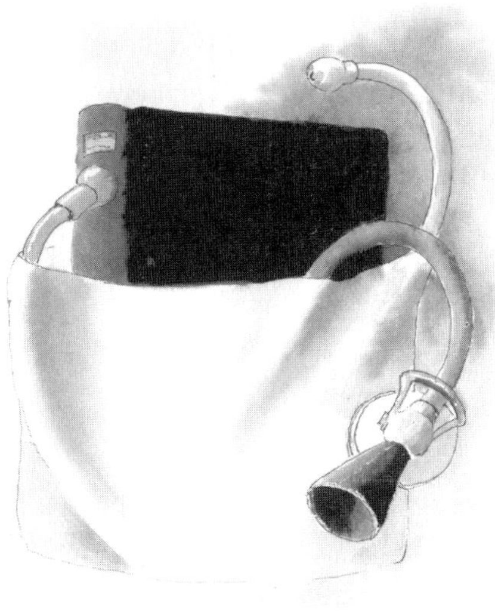

FINDING A ROOF

The good citizens of Dunedin have always considered their railway station to be a twin triumph of engineering and architecture. I failed to recognised this when I first stumbled onto its dimly lit platform in early March 1951. A cold, grey, wet blanket of an evening had already enveloped the place when the Christchurch - Invercargill express, after nine weary hours of travel, had jerked and hissed to a stop.

Reunited with my battered suitcase I passed through the brief warm glow of the waiting room to emerge onto the gloomy rain-swept taxi stand. A sharp chill in the air confirmed that after two days of travel I was indeed well south of Auckland.

One had been well advised. Arrive three days before first term, they said, and book into a student hostel while you seek accommodation more appropriate for those living on a government bursary.

The evening meal was nearly over when the taxi deposited me outside the hostel. A pleasant matronly figure welcomed me into the comfortable warmth of my temporary home and urged me to attend the dining room without delay. Obediently I pushed through the swing doors, joined the nearby queue and patiently advanced as the line contracted.

A subtle sense of unease quickly condensed into acute embarrassment. I was standing empty handed in the 'dirty dishes' queue where replete diners awaited their turn to scrape into a bucket those portions of the meal that lay beyond their requirements or had proved to be outside their gastronomic tolerance. Prompt reorientation directed me to the serving hatch which framed a tired yet gracious lady, not unlike my mother. She scanned me wearily while estimating my calorific capacity before depositing three dollops of food onto a warm plate - the classical meat and two veg.

Alone in the now empty dining room I contemplated the prosaic yet welcome meal. For the first time in my life I was a thousand miles from home.

The search for a more permanent roof began the next morning at the university lodgings office, a temporary facility established in a room marginally bigger than a broom cupboard and furnished with two chairs, a table and a telephone. On one of the chairs, like a gnome in a grotto, sat a small wrinkled man wearing a permanent frown folded above a pair of half-lens reading glasses.

Reluctantly he handed over addresses two at a time, scribbled on bits of paper. With them came the warning that each address must be checked out and one must be prepared to give good reasons for non-acceptance before further prospects would be released. Determined to be the model of responsibility I set forth.

A crowded tram sped me to the edge of the city and the end of the line. After a short walk I was face to face with the first offering. 143c was the middle unit of a series of five contiguous double story flats. A gap toothed, undulating picket fence struggled to contain the overgrown remnants of a long lost garden that fronted the property. Each unit was linked to the pavement by an uneven brick-paved path. A polished brass door knocker and gleaming letter flap promised close attention to cleanliness - which in Dunedin was Godliness.

The door was snatched open before my first hesitant tap could be joined by a second summons. Obviously my approach had been anticipated from within. The doorway was now filled by a middle aged woman whose generous proportions struggled to escape the confines of a blue and white check apron. The duster in her hand twitched nervously as she resisted dusting me down on the spot. The obligatory niceties were quickly disposed of and I was swept into the house with the artificial enthusiasm of a tour guide facing a three minute stop over.

Instead of pictures, the dark walls were punctuated with terse notes that demanded - WIPE YOUR SHOES - PLACE WET UMBRELLAS HERE - SWITCH OFF THIS LIGHT AFTER 9.30PM. The bathroom, a working memorial to exposed Edwardian plumbing, sported a coin operated, gas fired hot water cylinder. Alongside this a water-stained message reminded bathers to WIPE OUT AFTER USE. A similar missive on the toilet encouraged users to FLUSH AFTER USE.

The room on offer was upstairs, just beyond SILENCE AT ALL TIMES. A door labelled DON'T SLAM opened into a tiny room furnished with a small table, one chair and a bed. Disintegrating lace curtains failed to hide the uninspiring view of a brick wall beyond.

The prospect of months of study in this gloomy catacomb, surrounded by officious graffiti did not appeal. I was glad to escape with a vague promise to confirm later - and clicked the gate firmly behind me.

The second address was easily eliminated. A diminutive woman in her fifties peered through the half open door, scanned me in one sweep from head to foot and declared that the room had 'gorn' - before I could utter a word. As the door closed I was tempted to interject, "Don't slam".

The return journey was an event in itself. The empty tram hurtled along as though impatient to reach a long lost lover. The floor undulated in harmony with the uneven track while the sides swayed to their own unique intrinsic rhythm, even the seats constantly adjusted their shape as the stresses of the journey were transmitted through the inner structure of the vehicle. The effect suggested a double jointed hula dancer on fast forward. Everything that could move did so.

To take my mind off the perceived dangers inherent in this break-neck journey I contemplated my growing understanding of the business of student accommodation. Clearly it was orchestrated by middle aged people, many living outside the city boundary. They inhabited buildings just one step ahead of a demolition order (today any survivors probably boast a protection order). These folk radiated the same human warmth that one expected between a bomb and a bomb disposal expert. Even when defused by the house-rules, residents were merely tolerated as a necessary evil within the scheme of things. If home is where the heart is my heart was now desperate to return home.

Back at the university I found the lodgings office closed. The frowning gnome had gone to lunch and a small queue, which I promptly joined, had formed outside his grotto. By placing my need for shelter ahead of my desire for food I was making a statement which I hoped would be noted in my favour.

Standing in the queue and trying to ignore my hunger I slowly became aware of a familiar face moving into focus in front of me. It belonged to Walter - curly hair and glasses atop a shortish body and animated by eternal enthusiasm. We had met the previous evening at the hostel where he had observed my presence in the dirty dishes queue with restrained incredulity.

Presuming that I was still unhoused he informed me of a vacancy at his new found residence. If I hurried, he enthused, it could be mine - and only a brisk fifteen minute walk from the medical school.

With the address hastily recorded I thanked my new friend and made to depart. A hint of embarrassment clouded his face and, as I retreated, he asked hesitatingly, "By the way, are you Catholic?" "No", I assured him over my shoulder, and hurried away. I was anxious to reach 210 High Street before it to was 'gorn'.

TWO - ONE - OH

George Street divides Dunedin City into two contrasting halves. To the east, flat land reaches out to the wharves and the harbour beyond. Here one found the treasured railway station, light and not so light industry, the University and most of the city's slums - half of which belonged to the University and the other half to the Presbyterian Church.

To the west of George Street the land rises steeply, crumpled into hills and valleys. A band of trees, known affectionately as the Town Belt, marks the old city boundary. A better class of homes and most of the churches cling to these western hills. From here employers cast a benign eye over their workers who in turn look up to them. Within the scheme of things each had its place.

My course from the lodgings office lay southwards along George Street, past the best shops in town and through an eight sided mini-park known, with commendable logic, as the Octagon. Here a streaky-green statue of Robbie Burns is regularly acknowledged by the city bird life and largely ignored by its citizens.

A short distance beyond the Octagon, George Street is crossed by High Street and, together with some minor roads, creates a remarkably complex intersection known as The Exchange. Here, like an island in a river delta, an ornate memorial had been erected to the memory of Captain Cargill - a revered city father and onetime castle builder. Beneath this monument to past leadership lay a subterranean toilet for gentlemen. This curiously practical combination gave rise to the colourful euphemism "He's paying his respects to Cap'n Cargill", used by men to explain a fellow's temporary absence.

The level, eastern arm of High Street ran past the railway station. The western arm extended steeply upwards to the Town belt. This part of High Street was both high and very wide - wide enough to accommodate in its midline twin pairs of tracks for cable cars.

This service, which operated since 1881, was another Scottish engineering triumph. It shifted human tonnage with the same practical customer considerations commonly lavished on bags of wheat. The concept of adventure playgrounds began in High Street.

From early morning to late evening the vital cable ran continuously in a trench beneath the road's surface. The roof of this trench was split throughout its length by a central slot through which a keel-like structure extended down from the vehicle to grab or release the moving cable.

At each end of the cable car a tiny cabin sheltered six or so passengers and supported the roof that sheltered the rest of the structure. There were no sides. The driver stood in the middle and operated an impressive lever that simultaneously grabbed the cable and released the breaks, or vice versa.

Running fore and aft on either side of the driver was an elongated park bench that accommodated about a dozen sitting passengers. A further ten or so passengers (usually men) could stand on a foot plate, just beyond the seated travellers, forming a human curtain dangling precariously from overhead leather straps.

As I stood absorbing this curious phenomenon there was a sharp ding of a bell and the cable car jerked into motion and began its accent of High Street. On the footpath I followed in its wake in search of 210.

The steep footpath led past a couple of pubs and a few shops. With each step doubts began to gather. This was obviously a business area - an environment unlikely to offer shelter to students.

Suddenly there it was - 2.1.0. spelt out in gleaming brass. A double-storied brick building, encased in cement plaster, rose from the edge of the sloping footpath. A few concrete steps led to a formidable front door.

My timid summons was answered by a thirty - something woman who claimed, against the odds, to be the landlady. Her name was Meryl and she ushered me into a generous foyer furnished with an antique hall stand that offered pegs for coats and hats, a repository for umbrellas and a long mirror essential for pre-departure sartorial checks.

There wasn't a notice in sight. To the right a passageway led past various doors and ended in a large kitchen. To the left a flight of stairs ascended to the bedrooms.

The only room available was spacious and more than adequate for my needs. As a bonus a large window looked across the seried roofs of the city and snatched a glimpse of the harbour beyond. This was the room for me, although, at three pounds ten shillings a week for full board it was beyond my budget by about one pound. I hesitated, accepted and moved in. With five medical students in the place we had a mini student hostel on the very edge of the city.

As the day wore on fellow residents drifted in. Walter was first, still gently bubbling with enthusiasm. He introduced Graham, medium build, swarthy complexion and features that suggested a family tree with roots in Lebanon. Graham would be the cautious one. He would watch the small print for us and keep an eye on all the important dates in the University Calendar. Jim was the tall, quiet, introspective type, and, being the youngest kept his opinions to himself.

Dinner was on the table when Don arrived. His sense of timing, where meals were concerned, would become his trademark. Tall, solidly built and blondish, Don had the confidence that befitted his slight seniority.

Our first meal together was a pleasant family affair. As dining proceeded it became clear that for everyone present, including Meryl, this was a new experience. She had only recently taken over as landlady after separating from her husband. We were in fact her first lodgers, and over a cup of tea she nervously outlined the house rules. The ground floor rooms, excluding the kitchen, were her home and therefore no-go areas. The only telephone was in her sitting room and we could use this provided the sitting room door was open. A closed door signalled that she had visitors and did not wish to be disturbed.

With the rules in place, conversation lapsed until Graham raised the question - did anyone know where the nearest church was, and the times for Mass? A lively discussion followed as they explored the local distribution of services for catholics, leaving unbelievers such as Meryl and I standing on the sideline. I mentally withdrew and reflected on Walter's chance remark earlier in the day, suddenly seeing it in a new light. "Bill's not a Catholic", Walter observed quietly.

This announcement was received with a slight frown of collective disapproval and the subject was dropped leaving me feeling like a contaminant that had somehow entered an important experiment. Utopia had discovered its first flaw.

TWO SHORT WHITE COATS

Any hint of last night's religious miss-match had evaporated by next morning. Instead we were united by the common experience of our first day at Otago Medical School.

The morning was spent compiling time tables, book lists and inventories of essential equipment. At the top of everyone's list stood the entry "two short white coats". These would become a badge of office and a passport to all departments including, eventually, the hospital wards across the road. Stewards on the inter island ferry were the only other social group known to share our distinctive uniform!

This was the first time that all one hundred and twenty of us had come together. A mixed bag gathered from every corner of New Zealand. Some had served overseas during World War II and only one in twelve was a woman.

Despite our differences we all shared the relief and excitement that came with a seat in the school. We moved around the unfamiliar corridors like a well organised herd of zebras instinctively following a mysterious leader who somehow always knew where we should go next.

By midday the herd was heading for the watering hole - the student's common room - a long narrow room cluttered with chairs, tables, innumerable ash trays and dirty cups. Windows along one side gave out to the street and the hospital opposite. The place was already occupied by successful students from the previous year waiting alongside individual piles of books, bones and short white coats. The market was now open.

I found a beautiful set of bones, guaranteed to be complete and housed in a neat coffin-shaped wooden box. The vendor assured me that they were from India, female and aged about twenty five years. She served me well.

Saturday morning saw us introduced to the ritual of the Dissection Room. Here we would spend time over the next eighteen months wrestling with the mysteries of human anatomy supported by Gray's classic and other texts. Few of us had seen a dead human and yet we now faced the prospect of systematically cutting one into its component parts.

A sea of white coats had gathered in the corridor outside the closed double doors of the Dissection Room. The usual student gabble was reduced to a respectful murmur between anxious friends as we nervously faced this inevitable initiation, essential for further study.

The metallic click of the door bolts being withdrawn commanded a sudden silence. The doors were pushed open by a short father-like figure draped in a large brown dust coat. After a brief hesitation the class moved with a collective determination that disguised individual anxiety and we poured into a large white room furnished with ten tables.

On each table lay a body. The process of preservation had given a rich brown tan to the skin and all body hair was dyed red-brown. They were elderly (by our standards) and many had charred wounds. Rumour suggested that they may have been victims of the tragic fire at Seacliff Hospital some years previously.

By the time we had been divided up into ten groups of twelve (six for the left side of the body and six for the right) our noses had adjusted to the all pervading pong of formalin.

It was announced that our anatomy studies would begin in the arm pit (known in the trade as the axilla). Here we were destined to meet a fist full of nerves, blood vessels and muscles coming from whence we knew not and headed for destinations unknown. To me it seemed to be about as logical as beginning a study of music by attacking Beethoven's Ninth symphony half way through the second movement.

On the blackboard, directions for the first incision had been draughted with surgical precision and I had expected an enthusiastic rush from my fellows to grasp the scalpel and get on with it. Perhaps they had already decided on a career as school doctors and failed to hear the clarion call of surgery. I found myself the only one standing near the proffered axilla - everyone else had discovered some deeply absorbing item in their text books. Where I had anticipated competition there was none. With studied aplomp I took the knife (known in lay circles as a scalpel) and began the dissection.

I was surprised to find the fat to be golden and muscle tissue like corned beef - which of course was what we were dealing with here, anyway.

We soon learned that "our bod" was not exclusively ours at all. We would spend the year mining anatomical treasures from the shoulders to the feet. The head and neck belonged to the third year students and they would explore their territory during our absence at other studies.

We also had to adjust to visits between times by fifty dental students. Adapting to their presence in our medical school was a sensitive matter. To some they were seen as lesser beings but, none the less, it was prudent to be polite because if one failed to make a go of medicine one could always switch to dentistry. When facing the unknown a little prudence could be a wise move.

Today's medical students and graduates are more respectful towards their dental colleagues - addressing their personal dentist as 'sir' or 'ma-am' in the hope that such thoughtful expressions of respect will be reflected in more friendly professional fees.

Our introduction to the Dissection Room occupied the first Saturday morning at Medical School and by noon we were impatient to repair to the nearby Robbie Burns pub and review the morning's experiences over a pint.

In 1951 persons under twenty one (and most of us were) were deemed by law to be ineligible to consume alcohol on licenced premises. (Neither were we allowed to change gears in a taxi or cast a vote.). However I was assured that all bartenders in Dunedin were convinced that every student was 'of age'. As far as we were concerned anyone who had inhaled formalin for three hours had aged sufficiently. We ordered our first Dunedin beer with new confidence.

On this occasion drinking time for the 2.1.0 gang was limited. Meryl, mindful of our potentially stressful morning, had scheduled a cooked dinner for one p.m. After a couple of quick beers we hurried along now familiar George Street, where shops were closing, having completed their regulated Saturday morning's trade. Soon the streets would be empty until Monday morning, apart from sporadic activity around picture theatres on Saturday. This town, like every other town in New Zealand was doomed to die for a day and a half each week.

Although the morning had seen us initiated into the ultimate mystery of medical studenthood we were still bound to respond appropriately to the domestic imperative of being on time for meals - and we were.

The kitchen-dining room at 2.1.0 was dominated by an enormous, black, coal burning stove of indeterminate age, built by Shacklock of Dunedin - yet another engineering triumph. Our meal, ready for serving, lay in its warm womb of an oven.

Graham was the first to release an involuntary groan when Meryl opened the oven door and withdrew a plate of carved corned beef.

Missing the murmur of approval that every cook secretly anticipates when their morning's work is revealed, Meryl looked from one to the other of us searching for some sort of explanation. Don, true to form, was first to recover and helped himself to a generous serving of meat. Walter followed with contrived enthusiasm. Graham and Jim briefly contemplated a future as vegetarians. I was too hungry to brood on the irony of the situation - although I did compromise by cutting away the golden fat. Several days passed before anyone could explain to Meryl our hesitant response to that meal.

LAUNDRY BLUES

Saturday afternoons were dedicated to laundry duties. In this respect we bravely avoided the great tradition of Monday washday, making us the Seventh Day Adventists of laundry.

Since colonisation, New Zealanders had dedicated Mondays to the ritual cleansing of personal clothing and household linen. By mid morning every washhouse in the nation would be belching smoke as countless coppers struggled to boiling point. By lunchtime the more efficient housewife would have decked her washing line with dancing flags of whites and coloureds like bunting for a carnival. Cleanliness was alive, well, and fluttering in every backyard. Like justice it had to be seen to be done.

Our washhouse contained two wooden tubs surmounted by an ancient hand cranked wringer through which soggy clothes in one tub were squeezed across to the second. A brick encased, fire blackened copper dominated one corner, ready for the vital boil up.

The whole place was pervaded by a musty, earthy, slightly sour smell common to all washhouses with wooden tubs. This odour came from enzymes generated by micro-organisms that had colonised the wood. They broke down organic matter, including that which had soiled the clothes. Every housewife knew that an overnight soak in a smelly wooden tub did wonders for her whites and coloureds. Wooden tubs are now a matter of history and we buy our hungry enzymes in plastic packets. Progress is buying something we once had for free.

Unopposed I claimed the post of resident pyromaniac. (Hadn't I, at a very tender age, once set fire to two acres of gorse with only one match?). Furthermore I understood the iron-age technology of your average domestic copper and eventually had an impressive cloud of smoke and steam hanging from the rafters.

Periodically I would emerge from the heat and steam to carefully study the nature of the smoke rolling skywards from the chimney and then return to make fine adjustments to the draught. Onlookers were very impressed by this ritual - except Meryl, who knew that the damper mechanism had ceased to work long ago.

With the copper on a rolling boil, shavings carved from a bar of washing soap - manufactured on the flat land east of George Street - were dissolved in the turbulent water that was now ready to receive the week's wash. Distant echoes of a medieval witch's caldron haunted the scene.

At this stage the copper stick came into its own. This essential accessory was half the length of a broomstick and twice as thick. With it one prodded and stirred the copper's entangled contents and eventually hooked up individual items to transfer them, dripping and steaming, to the nearby tub of cold water where excess soapy water could be diluted. Any errant woollen item that had strayed into the copper was doomed to shrink to doll-like proportions.

From the cold water soak, items would be squeezed through the button-crunching wringer to a second tub of cold water, coloured with the dye methylene blue. A popular mantra 'out of the blue comes the whitest wash' was a national article of faith on wash-days. Today laundry consumption of this dye has significantly declined. In response, the enterprising marketers have convinced us to add the stuff to toilet cisterns where its mild antiseptic action gives domestic reassurance where none was necessary. However, a blue flush shows how much you really care.

From the 'blue' tub the wash would be squeezed via the button cruncher to a wicker basket and thence to the clothesline.

Exposing items of one's clothing to the frank gaze of others has a sobering effect - a gentle form of suburban exhibitionism. Sensitive housewives were known to conceal intimate items of clothing in pillow cases to protect the vulnerable from unbecoming thoughts. Lead us not into temptation - even on the washing line.

CHLOROPHYL

Although we still relied on Rekitt's Blue for the whitest wash, society was turning to science for solutions to the problems that dogged mankind. Users of Lifebouy Soap knew all about 'B.O.' and relied on this product simply because the soap stank more than the body ever could - the product lacked scientific subtlety.

The marketing breakthrough came with chlorophyl. Here was a natural substance everyone recognised from school science and it was a simple matter to con the public into believing that this wonder of the plant kingdom not only could produce oxygen but could also destroy odours.

Within a matter of weeks every brand of toothpaste, every gargle and mouthwash and all wick deodourisers contained miraculous green chlorophyl. Failure to use these new products came close to personal negligence. One bookseller in George Street picked up on the fad by filling his shop window with dictionaries appropriately arranged beneath a large notice which read;
"ALL THESE BOOKS CONTAIN CHLOROPHYL."

The great chlorophyl swindle collapsed as quickly as it had appeared - encouraged no doubt by some wag who wrote;
"The goat you smell on yonder hill has grazed all day on chlorophyl."

Suddenly toothpaste was white again.

AN ANONYMOUS BENEFACTOR

Life settled into an inflexible rhythm of days of lectures and nights of study. On Sunday mornings the others went to Mass, Meryl slept in and I cooked breakfast. It was a comfortable time marred slightly by the nagging reminder that I could not afford to stay longer than one term.

Each day, in the student common room, I persued further investigations into the state of accommodation in Dunedin and soon realised that all suitable placements were now occupied.

Those who could afford it were comfortably established in student hostels. A lucky few had found board in private homes where they were treated like long lost sons or daughters and spoilt rotten. Some late-comers had found themselves saddled with embittered, middle aged landladies and were already desperate for a merciful release. (In the student vernacular these women were known as "twenty watt landladies" in recognition of the restrictions they imposed on lighting for study.) Most senior students and a few juniors had moved into flats, which, then as know, were usually substandard structures in various states of decay awaiting demolition and redevelopment.

Flatting was very strictly a single-sex affair. The University Senate demanded standards of moral behaviour that, if breached, could lead to prompt expulsion. In this respect medical and theology students seemed to share the greatest risk of censure.

A group of senior colleagues quickly learned how vulnerable their grip on tertiary education could be. One of their number had a sister who shared a flat across town with other women. Their laundry facilities for some reason were temporarily inoperable and could she use her brother's equipment? By Saturday afternoon the boy's clothesline was sporting various items of female attire. By Monday morning the boys were in the Dean's office where an explanation was demanded and only reluctantly accepted.

The presence of sweet eccentricity among us can be the spice that lifts our daily lives and colours social interaction but it can sometimes overwhelm, like too much curry, tainting life's repast. One could describe Ned as eccentric. He lived in a world uniquely his own. A world where conformity was anathema.

He, and a few student mates, occupied an upstairs flat which was faithfully mirrored by an identical unit down stairs, occupied by some disapproving young ladies.

One of Ned's peculiar habits centred around his attitude to washing. He approached this subject with a spirit of conservation towards both effort and materials that anticipated today's concern against waste - but he carried it to extreme.

Every Saturday night he washed - everything. Ned would fill the bath and dump into it the week's dirty clothes and then, fully dressed, would climb in as well. With a golden bar of trusty Sunlight Soap he would scrub the shirt he wore, remove it, and proceed in this way until he was naked. He then washed Ned before turning his attention to the flotsam of dirty clothes still suspended in the grey soup that now surrounded him.

In the bathroom directly below, the ladies also observed the national tradition of Saturday night baths.

One of Ned's flat mates, aware of the synchronised bathing habits and endowed with a working knowledge of physics, hydrodynamics and plumbing, had an idea. Armed with a handful of old rag he sneaked around the back of the building and stuffed the rag plug tightly up the drainpipe that served both units and waited for Ned to pull the plug. The very grubby waste water thus released hurtled down the pipe, impacted on the obstruction and surged back, driving a considerable volume of trapped air ahead of it. This sudden back-pressure lifted the bath plug in the down stairs flat releasing a cascade of violent, obscene bubbles followed by a vigorous jet of very off-colour water that now snaked around the bath and the very startled bather.

On the following Monday morning we received the account of this prank with great hilarity. The fact that we did so says something about the immature relationships that existed between the sexes. The 'them and us' thing tainted humour in those days in a way that underlined masculine insecurity.

On the other hand, even today the scene would raise a laugh in a sit-com.

I was not the only one at 2.1.0 living on a bursary yet it appeared I was the only one faced with the need to consider cheaper accommodation. If they could manage, why couldn't I? As weeks passed my sense of incompetent financial management increased. Although I had no alternative placement arranged I felt I should warn Meryl of my coming need to relocate.

Meryl was alone in the kitchen when I raised the matter. It transpired that she also wanted to discuss the same subject and had news for me. Did I know that the others were subsidised to the tune of one pound per week by an anonymous catholic benefactor? Furthermore that same person was prepared to support me by the same amount.

Suddenly I could see why the others managed when I was struggling. One mystery dissolved and a new one crystallised. The question now was, should I accept? I could hear my mother's voice. "Beggars can't be choosers." I accepted.

For days I was elated by the prospect of staying, though at times I worried about how to express my gratitude to the mysterious, benevolent Catholic who had extended such kindness to a Protestant, albeit a lapsed one.

My acceptance created a new bond with my fellow residents. Although we did not share religious convictions we now enjoyed common sponsorship. The identity of our supporter was a frequent topic of conversation in which Meryl steadfastly refused to assist us.

Meryl's most frequent visitor was a chap called Chris. He was fortyish, short, stocky, quietly spoken and always in a hurry. From time to time Chris would appear like a genie, usually in the afternoon and evaporate before tea. The odds were that if the sitting room door was shut, Chris was visiting. Occasionally Meryl would leave him behind the closed door and get on with whatever household duties were pressing at the time.

Eventually he was recognised with his family at church - establishing yet another connection with the all embracing Catholic faith. He was even briefly entertained as the anonymous benefactor.

It was Graham's aunt who cracked the mystery. She lived in Dunedin and regularly gave hospitality to her nephew. On this occasion they were standing on the steps of 2.1.0 when Chris emerged, greeted Graham, politely raised his hat to auntie and promptly disappeared down High Street.

"Who's that?" she asked.

"Chris, a friend of Meryl's."

"Looks like a bookie to me!" she replied.

Inside Graham's head things suddenly fell into place and we were promptly summoned to a meeting in his room.

"Think about it. When is he here? Saturdays, Wednesdays and occasional holidays - all of them race days somewhere in the country. And what does a bookie need? A radio and a telephone somewhere that is safe - and what could be safer from the cops than a boarding house full of unworldly, cashstrapped students and if all of this is true, then right now we are living in a den of iniquity that could be raided any minute."

The level of anxiety rose with each new observation, reaching a crescendo when the final connection was made. Chris was our benefactor. Instead of paying rent for the use of the place, thereby incriminating Meryl, he was making an anonymous donation that could not be traced.

At first the others felt cheated - but I didn't. After all, my inclusion in his expenses was over and above the agreement we presumed he had struck with Meryl.

Someone pointed out that at law we were being supported through proceeds of illegal gambling - a prospect that greatly worried Graham. He could now see us in court, swearing on a stack of Bibles to tell the truth, the whole truth and nothing but.

Our mutually generated tension was at bursting point when we surged downstairs to confront Meryl with the labyrinthine logic that had entangled us in the past half hour. She quietly agreed with our analysis and then brought everyone down to earth by asking if anyone, in the light of this revelation, wished to leave?

Righteous indignation was suddenly smothered by common sense. Life as a student at 2.1.0 was too good, (and too affordable) to be overturned by concern for a law that made it illegal to bet on a horse outside the boundaries of a race-course.

Shortly after auntie's observation we were back to normal. A pity about the mysterious benefactor, but if Chris chose to pay his rent by subsidising ours - then lucky us. Necessity mothered yet another invention. We promptly invented a passionate concern for the punter who chose to support private enterprise. In order to save the Dean unnecessary concern for our moral standing we agreed to keep the true identity of 2.1.0 to ourselves.

The following year, when the law was toughened, making a jail sentence mandatory for all bookies and their retainers (thus preparing the ground for T.A.B off course betting) Chris declared that no one would be imprisoned because of his chosen livelihood. He promptly retired from the scene and took up selling life insurance.

The end of Chris' days as a bookie saw the end of our subsidy. We responded by turning 2.1.0 into a flat. Meryl, who had had enough of cooking and cleaning, secured a job as a tram conductor, happily gathering fares and clanging bells as she hurtled and swayed across the city.

Technically, of course, we had created a mixed flat and every week our washing line bore silent witness to this fact. Our vulnerability in the new circumstances simply was not mentioned. High walls hid the tell-tale line from vindictive view and within the walls of 2.1.0 we continued our innocent co-existence.

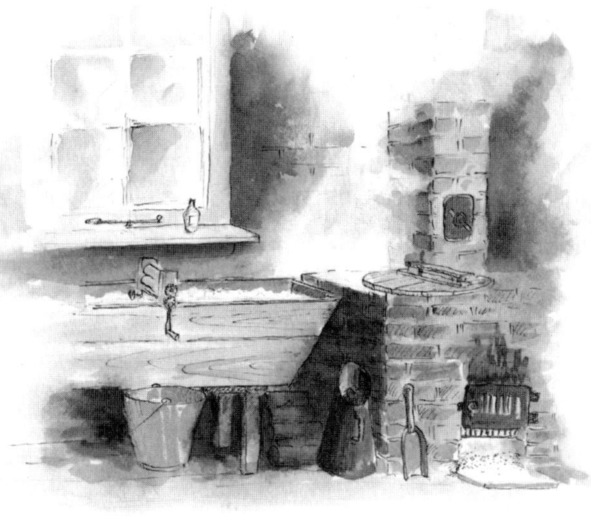

Wash day 2.1.0

CROSSING THE ROAD

For eighteen months our study focussed steadfastly on the academic. We were taught the normal human everything – normal anatomy, normal physiology and normal biochemistry while we gazed longingly across the road to the hospital where fascinating abnormality ruled. Furthermore, each teaching department independently assumed that their subject occupied the epicentre of the medical world and any inter-relationship with other subjects was a regrettable aberration.

Teaching standards were alarmingly uneven. Although our tutors and lecturers were recognized leaders within their fields, this did not, of itself make them good communicators. A weak link in the system was the traditional appointment of postgraduate researchers as junior lecturers without regard to their teaching skills, in order to give them a modest income. In some subjects we learned far more from textbooks than from lectures and tutorials.

A notable exception to this criticism was Bill Adams, Professor of Anatomy. He could convey the complicated sequences of embryonic development with enchanting lucidity. He also possessed a legendary photographic memory that earned him universal respect. At our first lecture he called the roll with slow deliberation, looking up to identify each respondent, then mentally snapping their image into his personal I.D. system, thus logging all one hundred and twenty of us into his memory bank. Subsequently he would rattle through the names while simply listening to the cadence of our responses. Any attempt to answer for an absent friend would promptly register as a fault in the system – the name would be repeated, silence would prevail and the absence solemnly noted. Bill's lectures always enjoyed full attendance.

Although written exams had been accepted as a way of life since secondary school days this school had a new experience on offer which they dignified with the arcane title 'Viva Voce' and we called 'orals'. We viewed this novel concept with about the same enthusiasm as a prisoner would on hearing about new facilities in the torture chamber.

For orals we were required to dress 'professionally' (men a suit), and one by one sit in front of an examiner to answer questions. Should you find yourself confronting a junior lecturer the chances were that you had passed the written paper. Facing the professor suggested you were either destined for honours or were in imminent danger of failing.

It would take a couple of weeks for the class to complete orals and for the examiners to assemble the results. For some obscure bureaucratic reason the University of New Zealand ruled that it must confirm all professional examination passes before they could be announced and this would take weeks to process. The Medical School, though bound by the dictum, proceeded, with characteristic cunning, to short – circuit this potential hiatus by releasing, not the passes – but the failures.

It was a strange experience to stand in a draughty, empty foyer scanning a notice entitled 'The following have *failed* to satisfy the examiners,' while desperately praying that your name would not appear.

Having successfully satisfied the First Professional examiners we now stood poised to cross Great King Street – the boundary separating the school from the hospital – the normal human from the abnormal and the academic from the clinical. Now was the time to pack up our bones and books and prepare to flog them off to next year's innocent intake.

Rites of passage demand symbols of proof and the icon we now sought was the stethoscope. Fortunately this tell – tale, surrogate identity badge defied concealment. Tucked modestly in a pocket of our short white coats it could be safely relied on to uncoil like a snake in a basket revealing its presence to all. If the ability to build a compact, concealable stethoscope existed the market for it certainly did not.

FROM PROFESSIONAL ICON TO FASHION ACCESSORY

Even our treasured symbol, the stethoscope, was destined to lose its exclusive and unique association with our chosen profession. Physicians have always been the most dedicated of all to this curious contraption - and consultant physicians more than others. Consultants rarely wore white coats, thus placing themselves clearly above and beyond the white-uniformed retinue that followed them in solemn procession around the wards. These be-suited leaders carried their personal stethoscopes coiled in their hands rather like the country squire authoritatively gripping a riding crop while addressing the peasants. It conveyed a sense of power with a hint of discipline. (Anyway their tailors strictly forbade them to pocket the thing for fear of spoiling the fit of their jackets.)

Surgeons were less in awe of the stethoscope and often did not carry one, preferring to borrow from members of their respectful retinue. They would casually accept the icon pointing out that it was not so much the instrument that counted but what went between the earpieces when it was used.

The discovery of drugs able to treat hypertension began the erosion of the status previously enjoyed by the stethoscope. Our Professor of Medicine, Sir Horace Smirk, was a leader in this field and in order to obtain an extensive series of blood pressure readings from a ward full of patients he engaged lay people to monitor the patient's response and progress. Each of these new comers to the ward carried a stethoscope. Not to be outdone it wasn't long before nurses followed suit and the inexorable devaluation of this icon was established.

The profession had always followed an inflexible tradition with respect to the correct wearing of stethoscopes. During an examination, but when not actually in use, the instrument should hang from the neck via the gently embracing arms of the earpieces so that the chest attachment dangled at about umbilical level. The disdainful, new-comer Philistines quickly adopted the foreign practice of wearing the thing draped around their necks like the common university scarf, with the chest piece to the left and the ear attachments draped casually on the right. (Reverse for left handers.) As access to this instrument spread to paramedics and other lesser beings, this shameful habit spread upwards until it is now universal and followed by all participants in today's hospital dramas - with the exception, of course, of the Consultants.

The gentle, all pervading euphoria that followed the simple crossing of a street, armed with an undisciplined stethoscope, was as sweet as it was short lived. Within the multi-layered hierarchy of a teaching hospital we soon learned how close we stood to the untouchables. The Consultant (referred to in yesteryear as an 'Honorary' because they then gave their time to the hospital without fee) besuited, aloof and ever anxious to return to the 'rooms' where the real money lay, stood unchallenged at the top. Next, the Junior Specialists followed by Senior Registrars and Registrars down to the humble, harassed, overworked Housesurgeon. Senior nursing staff stood somewhere between Registrars and Housesurgeons while medical students occupied a vague zone just above hospital porters but differed from them in that porters were actually needed within the scheme of things.

In every hospital the nursing staff occupied and administered a second hierarchy of organized power. At its head stood the Matron – the archetypical authority figure who would float through the establishment on a cloud of entrenched, tightly ordered respect, before disappearing into her office to drink tea from delicate bone china cups and arrange the invitation list for the next Nurses' Ball. She was as close to royalty as any commoner could aspire and all nursing staff when addressed by her, would stand erect with both hands respectfully clasped behind their backs. The hint of a curtsy would not be out of place. The Mother Superior of the bedpan, replaced today by a Nursing Manager armed with a pocket calculator – a transition regretted by romantics but not universally mourned by the modern nurse.

Ward Sisters were to their wards what the Matron was to the entire hospital. These women (all spinsters), once appointed to a ward, would usually complete their professional lives married to that task, their names often becoming synonymous with their territory.

In common with their supreme commander, Ward Sisters wore a veil on their heads

– a square of starched white fabric, somewhat bigger than a table napkin. At a distance and with the light behind her, her veil became the closet thing to a halo one could find in western culture since the renaissance painters.

In our time many Ward Sisters had served overseas as nurses to the armed forces during the Second World War. Their knowledge of the management of trauma, shock and pain often exceeded that of the medical teams they now worked alongside. Students and Housesurgeons learned a lot from these women. Many senior nurses had been engaged to soldiers whose names were eventually carved in granite on memorials scattered through the country. In bitter, silent sorrow many dedicated themselves subsequently to a lifetime of service to nursing.

Nursing was based on a unique female monastic order that was as restrictive in many ways as the religious orders of antiquity. All nurses, from student to Matron, were required to 'live in' in the Nurses' Home. Marriage automatically terminated most nursing careers and pregnancy outside marriage brought prompt, unconditional expulsion.

Together with minimum pay all nurses received their uniforms, meals and a bed in a tiny cell. Nobody could absent themselves without a leave pass. Parents (particularly country folk) saw nursing as the safest path for their daughters to take on that hazardous journey between puberty and marriage. A steady stream of applicants eager to enter the profession was thereby guaranteed.

Within a few years this apparently solid structure would begin to erode as businesses and organizations outside the state hospital system offered work to trained nurses irrespective of their marital state or place of residence. As the stock of senior nurses began to shrink, hospital based nursing would be forced to face the new challenge, eventually exposing the real cost of nursing services. Nursing education, once an exclusive function if hospitals, would be moved to tertiary institutions and eventually Nurses' Homes would become empty monuments.

Entry into the wards gave us access to a captive audience – patients. Their state of capture was endorsed by their uniform – ill fitting hospital night attire worn for the duration of their indefinite stay in a dormitory shared with about twenty others. Their personal stake consisted of a bed, a locker and a chair. Occasionally, an illusion of privacy from the curious passing parade might be offered by a series of hastily erected folding screens.

Despite all this they were indeed patient – and gracious with it. To refer to them as 'clients' would have been ridiculous. 'Patients,' conditioned by their circumstances, gratefully accept without question whatever is on offer. 'Clients' expect to have a say in everything, knowing that one way or the other they have paid for it, or are about to do so.

Our first task in the wards was to gain experience in taking case histories but as we were about the sixth person to lead them through their story the experience had lost something of its novelty. None the less the patient's day was long and featureless so that chatting to a student, and thereby contributing to the education of future doctors, had something to commend it.

By now they knew exactly which symptoms to emphasize and some, who had gained a special insight into their malady, were able to offer an in-depth analysis of the underlying pathology. Although appreciated, this tended to undermine the real objective of the exercise.

It is humbling to realize how much our education relied on the generosity of others – from making their dead bodies available for dissection to sharing the private details of their lives. Will the day come when all this is given a dollar value? I hope not.

One's first patient, like one's first day in the dissection room, is always remembered. Mine taught me a lot even though we did not share a common language. He was a middle aged Iranian merchant seaman who had vomited a vast amount of blood from an inoperable stomach cancer. He had received a few pints of Christian blood, his ship had sailed and he lay dying in a foreign land isolated by language, religion, culture and geography.

Armed with a pocket compass and an atlas, together we established the direction of Mecca which comforted him a little, while I learned that when the scope of medicine was exceeded and 'nothing more could be done' there was still room for humanity.

As part of our orientation within the hospital we were conducted through the various departments like so many tourists. Our visit to the X Ray Department, however, was quite a highlight. Here we were proudly shown their latest acquisition – a fluoroscope. This consisted of a vertical screen large enough to cover an entire person standing behind it. In a darkened room X-rays were shot through the subject projecting their skeleton onto the screen with a chilling yellow – green glow.

When the call for volunteers fell upon deaf ears a couple of students were selected at random to take turns behind the screen. It was a bit of a giggle to see their bones together with coins in their pockets and other metallic accessories included in the display.

Suddenly, while watching this innocent projection of bones and metal, a wave of intense nausea flooded through me. That very morning one of my fly buttons had slipped its moorings and I had resorted to a safety pin to effect temporary repairs. There, but for the Grace of God, I could now be standing, stupidly displaying my lax house keeping to the entire class and half the X-ray staff.

At this time fluoroscopes also enjoyed a brief popularity in shoe stores where a foot sized version was used to display the comfortable disposition of foot bones within a new shoe – to the delight of kids, customers and the store staff. They were suddenly withdrawn (along with the hospital version) when their capacity to scatter lethal rays was established.

THINGS THEATRICAL

I discovered, buried within the bowels of the hospital, a windowless wonderland where miracle plays with varying casts were enacted daily. Furthermore, seats in the dress circle were free.

The Americans lost something when they named places for surgery 'Operating Rooms' - the O.R. This mundane title failed to acknowledge the unique nature of the performances staged therein. The Brits, on the other hand, recognizing the drama involved, chose the word 'Theatre' instinctively.

The surgeon invariably starred the show which usually co-starred the Theartre Sister and included occasional direction from the Anaesthetist. A variable cast, mainly of nurses, would appear as chorus and extras. Each day a programme entitled "Theatre List" would be posted enabling students and others to choose the event with the most promise. Patient's names always received billing on the list but for all practical purposes they functioned as essential props and were rarely given speaking parts.

Theatres in teaching hospitals had an upstairs viewing platform from which students could view the proceedings in the hope of learning something from the performance. An inclined plateglass barrier protected both the patient and surgical team from any debris that might threaten the overall cleanliness of the scene below.

There was a wonderful freedom associated with the whole business. Students could attend the viewing area as they pleased and from time to time they could be invited as extras to come down and assist. Assisting consisted of masking, scrubbing up and gowning so that you could stand in the same position for an hour or so numbly hanging onto a retractor while desperately trying to keep out of the way. This was one of the few places were the nursing staff welcomed the involvement of students. With enough of them swinging on retractors the nurses could get away to lunch on time.

We soon learned that being attached to a retractor would not significantly advance a future in surgery. At best you gained an occasional glimpse into the wound, but for most of the time were left to contemplate the back of the surgeon's head.

Despite the ever present potential for drama, most operations were boring. Occasionally the anaesthetist would punctuate the proceedings with little bursts of repartee induced, according to legend, to a long association with the disinhibiting properties of anaesthetic gasses.

During the recent war years many consultants had been encouraged, on patriotic grounds, to re-enter hospital service or delay their retirement. This eventually left many hospitals with a significant number of older practitioners - particularly surgeons. Some of these had learned their basic surgery on the battlefields of the Great War where speed in amputating limbs was the accepted indicator of surgical skill.

Two events from my student theatrical experiences remain firmly etched in my memory. The first involved an elderly surgeon of the old school who was scheduled to perform a prostatectomy. In those days this was a risky procedure performed through the lower abdomen in the space between the bladder and the pubic bone - a deep narrow cave in which one fumbled blindly in a pool of blood to shell out the offending organ.

Now this old chap had two grudges. He disparaged anaesthetists and hated women doctors. That day he found himself rostered on with a double outrage - a woman anaesthetist.

On this occasion the anaesthetist upstaged the surgeon. She was proudly using the hospital's latest anesthetic machine and enthusiastically demonstrating its dials and spinning gas flow bobbins to a gaggle of attentive students.

Slowly the rich, red ooze of blood welling up from the wound began to darken and eventually turn black. With a gesture of disgust the surgeon stripped off his gloves and leaned over to growl in her ear, "My end's just died – how's yours? "Theatre erupted into a flurry of activity but in the end both ends died.

My second theatre anecdote also involved the introduction of new equipment but this time has a happier outcome.

It was soon after "Reader's Digest" had published an article on the new-fangled 'Bloodless Electric Knife' that Dunedin Hospital purchased one. This device, known as diathermy, was really a miniature electric welding kit which generated a hot little spark at the tip of a small blunt blade. With this blade the surgeon could cut tissue and seal off small blood vessels at the same time. Diathermy was recommended for many operations including the removal of piles and it was for this procedure that the shiney new machine was proudly wheeled into the surgical area.

Appropriately draped and fully anaesthetized the patient lay on his back with legs spread-eagled. The young surgeon, standing between the legs, liberally swabbed the exposed area to sterilize the skin. Nervously he picked up the electrode, pressed on the foot pedal and struck the first spark.

There was a muffled 'boom' and a blue flame danced briefly above the exposed genitalia. In the shocked silence that followed the anaesthetist leaned forward and in a stage whisper that all could hear observed, "That's the worst case of bare faced arson I have ever seen."

Later that day the theatre sister made a note to omit methylated spirits for skin preparation when they next used diathermy.

PASSING GAS

The ability to render a patient unconscious while a surgeon cut them up was a skill expected of all doctors by the time they were fully registered. The art of anaesthetics belonged in the realm of general practice and hospitals relied on local G.P.s to provide this service. There was no way Dunedin Hospital could train one hundred and twenty students each year in this field so by default it was left to most of us to explore the subject during our first post graduate year.

We did, however, experience fleeting contact with the business of ether anaesthesia during a short stint in the E.N.T. Department where it was the preferred agent during tonsillectomy in children. Indeed, since 1846 ether had retained its popularity as an anaesthetic vapour despite its disconcerting capacity to form explosive mixtures with air. There was a time in the mid nineteenth century that well to do young adults indulged in 'ether frolics' where the participants reached various levels of intoxication after inhaling the vapour.

In about 1800 nitrous oxide (laughing gas) had been shown by Sir Humphry Davy to reduce response to pain but when used alone this gas failed to provide the depth of effect necessary for most operations, although dentists found it useful.

Because it did not form explosive mixtures with air, chloroform had enjoyed brief favour as an anaesthetic agent (particularly in Obstetrics) until its capacity to rot livers and cause sudden death lead to its fall from grace.

With a track record stretching back over a century ether still held its place although its administration called for a gentle persuasive touch. One of our anaesthetic tutors summed up the technique for us during a tonsil session. His analogy would fail today's requirement for political correctness but was none the less useful and readily memorable. Isn't that what all good teaching should be?

He suggested that we approach the subject the same way we would pursue a little romantic flirtation. First we were to be clear about our goal and sustain a determination to reach it. We should introduce the vapour lightly and casually and just as casually ease up should the advance be resisted, then, just as gently return to our purpose with a little more ether on the mask. With each breath compliance would increase leading inevitably to ultimate success.

Anaesthesia for adults was undergoing significant changes. The intravenous barbiturate Pentothal had rendered vaporous sedation redundant. With Pentothal, sleep was quick, pleasant and unresisted. The anaesthetist's trolley was now hung about with various gas bottles, each painted distinctive colours for identification and each topped by suitable gauges that lead to flow metres and thence to a face fitting mask.

For a while even carbon dioxide was added to the selection in the belief that it would stimulate respiration in those patients disinclined to breath deeply. The gas cyclopropane enjoyed brief acceptance as an anaesthetic agent around this time but it disappeared from the trolley almost as quickly as it appeared. One of my mentors summed up its dangers in one unforgettable phrase - "Remember my boy - with this stuff they always die pink".

We were among the last of the profession expected to be able to administer an anaesthetic simply because we were doctors. Today G.P. Anaesthetists continue to provide a valued service in this field and treat the subject as the specially it has become. However most major anaesthetics are now give by full time specialists.

Most of the great advances in surgery that have been achieved in the last half of this century were made possible by developments in the art and science of anaesthesia. Surgeons can perform miracles for as long as the anaesthetist can keep the patient alive.

A LEGACY OF VENUS

Diseases that we called venereal (from Venus, the Roman goddess of love) are today banally referred to as 'sexually transmitted diseases'. Thus poetry is consumed by pragmatism.

Every hospital associated with a shipping port has been obliged for decades to offer a free clinic for all visiting sailors (and their shore bound local contacts) who had reason to believe that they may be suffering from a sexually transmitted disease. We called these outposts of fear and desperation V.D. (Venereal Disease) Clinics and the clinician in charge was traditionally refered to as the 'pox doctor'. The derision that tainted this title ignored the riches that came with the possession of a confidential private consultant service to an anxious public. Folk who usually scorned payment for medical services were always willing to reconsider when it came to the delicate personal issue of V.D.

Our tutors emphasized the importance of seeing and eventually recognizing the early sores of syphilis and urged us to watch the shipping news published in the Otago Daily Times. The incubation period of syphilis, it transpired, was about the same as the time it took the banana boat to sail from Fiji to Dunedin. Apparently with each fresh supply of bananas you could count on at least one new patient at the hospital clinic. I never resorted to the shipping news - but gave up on bananas for several years.

If the banana boat failed to deliver, one could always resort to the Pathology Museum where a large glass jar containing a human head suspended in murky preservative was on show. This insensitive exhibit nicknamed "Sinbad the Sailor", taught a little about syphilitic lesions and a lot about the values of the time. I hope it was removed long ago and disposed of with appropriate dignity.

Dunedin's prosperous private V.D. clinic was in High Street, opposite and a little below our residence of 2.1.0. From our top floor we commanded a good view of the building – a substantial private residence identified only by its street number. There were two entrances. One lead to the front door while a side driveway curved around to the back. The patients, each with a carefully timed appointment, presented themselves singly at the unlit front door and emerged later via the tradesman's entrance (quite appropriately in some cases) to melt anonymously into the night. The clinic functioned three times a week – always half an hour after dark.

In the few years since penicillin had been available the incidence of both syphilis and gonorrhea had begun to decline from the high levels encountered during World War Two.

Syphilis takes its name from a character in the play 'Syphilis Sive Morbus Gallicus' (Syphilis the French Disease) published in 1530 by a Veronese Physician. The French retaliated by suggesting that Columbus and his crew brought it back as a present from the American Indians. However, in the interest of international harmony, there is a strong theory that syphilis was in Europe long before Columbus but it was confused with leprosy, giving rise to the false belief that leprosy was highly contagious (especially through sexual contact). It was also known at the time that some cases of 'Leprosy' responded to the application of mercury – which is correct for syphilis but not for genuine leprosy. Indeed mercury was the only practical treatment for syphilitic sores until 1909 when Salvarsan offered more hope.

Treating syphilis with mercury gave rise to the corny old adage 'spend one night with Venus and the rest of your life with Mercury'.

FREE DELIVERY

Part of our obstetrics training obliged us to attend and record in detail the progress and outcome of a dozen deliveries. To facilitate this five of us at a time were granted temporary residence in a suite of tiny cells adjacent to the delivery rooms in the Dunedin Hospital Maternity Unit. Here we experienced our first taste of being 'on call' day and night - a pattern that for many of us would be a way of life in the years to come.

The unit consistently operated at, or just beyond, peak capacity for most of the time. Only a few years earlier thousands of men had returned from the war to fall into the welcoming arms of their womenfolk. Child bearing was by now a national duty and the post-war baby boom was indeed booming.

In 1939 the first Labour Government had established free maternity care and hospital delivery throughout the land. Home delivery, the norm for previous generations, had evaporated like the morning mist and midwives now only functioned within the shelter of a hospital. To expect a home birth in the fifties bordered on negligence.

Prior to 1939 childbirth had been an expensive business. As a pre-schooler I was aware that a man called regularly at our home and received a coin from my mother. He would solemnly record this transaction in a book before departing. I eventually learned that she was still paying for my entry into this world some four years after the event - and we were the lucky ones. My parents had been classified as 'deserving poor' and my birth had been partly subsidised through Charitable Aid.

Women who now laboured under Labour did so in state maternity hospitals with National Womens' Hospital in Auckland as their flagship. Here standards were set for the whole of New Zealand and women whose pregnancies were in any way complicated could confidently expect state of the art advice, supervision and management.

Those blessed with a normal healthy pregnancy however were regarded as rather boring and in a way less deserving of the elaborate facilities available. Their labour and subsequent delivery often proceeded with the same understanding and consideration that Henry Ford lavished on the production of motor cars.

The organised efficiency of the factory was more apparent than real, especially when the number in labour exceeded the capacity of the system to accommodate them. Under these circumstances women on the verge of delivery found themselves lined up in their beds like so many laden ships desperate to enter port. The command 'pant don't push' implied that the mother soon-to-be could now spontaneously resume control and responsibility over an event that neither she nor the staff in these circumstances could manage. The long anticipated 'blessed event' became a chaotic blur where nature invariably triumphed over human ingenuity.

The only males admitted to this inner sanctum of parturition were doctors - or in our case students. A visitor from outer space would have concluded that human reproduction was at best immaculate or at least parthenogenic.

Chain smoking husbands (the only partner recognised by the system was through marriage) were confined to a waiting room suitably remote from the action. Here they wandered restlessly, each enveloped in a private personal mixture of guilt and remorse as they contemplated their contribution to the anxious state of affairs. Most of them accepted their exclusion from the birth with a profound relief that nourished the attitude among men that babies were women's business and best left that way. The relationship between father and child thus began with a significant disadvantage.

The first delivery I attended was a disaster for all concerned and still haunts me. The experience forced me to seriously reconsider – albeit briefly – my choice of profession.

The babe had been shown on X Ray to be grossly deformed and was believed to have died during the early stages of labour. The task was to deliver a large abnormal foetus that would eventually emerge still - born. Painfully slowly the misshapened babe, its giant head clamped firmly in obstetric forceps, slipped out, followed closely by the placenta. The entire mass, caught up in a white drape, was lowered into a bucket at the foot of the table while attention focussed on the exhausted, grieving, bleeding mother.

After a few seconds the babe gave three of four shallow gasps and then surrendered its tenuous claim to life. This erratic and belated attempt to breath changed the situation to neonatal death and not the still-birth that everyone, including the mother, expected. However the outcome was the same and a sad little bundle was wisked away to the sluice room.

For a long time I wondered about the ultimate fate of that pathetic parcel and eventually learned that the practice at the time involved a junior nurse who would have been instructed to convey the 'products of conception' to the hospital boiler house and to personally supervise its placement in the furnace. Having observed its despatch she would return to the delivery suite office and sign for her task in a book kept for that purpose.

In some parts of the country local undertakers sometimes offered an alternative free service whereby a still-born babe would be concealed in the next coffin due for burial. This practice could be seen as marginally preferable to the casual destruction, along with hospital waste, in the boiler furnace but of course it raised new questions involving two families now linked unknowingly in their separate grief.

The hospital based maternity machine certainly included efficiencies that contributed to lowered rates of early infant deaths, but it was unable to respond sensitively and sensibly to those events that still remained beyond its control. Any still-born babe or neonatal death that occurred in spite of our best efforts was seen as a profound and embarrassing failure that had to be swept away before it eroded everyone's confidence in an obviously flawed system. The parent's right, in these circumstances, to be involved and to grieve, simply was not part of the equation. In effect we operated within a dictatorship that would persist for several decades before repeated challenges could restore a more human face. Ironically National Women's Hospital would be among the first to fall from grace.

CAUSES OF DEATH

Of all the departments that set out to teach us, the Pathology Department had the most problems and the least success in solving them. Pathologists have several limitations when it comes to organising teaching sessions. Whereas the physicians and surgeons have wards full of cases to choose from, the poor old pathologists have to wait until someone dies and even then they only have the body for a day or so.

Non the less they always have the last say and take a perverse pride in demonstrating the accuracy or otherwise of the diagnosis, previously entered by their medical or surgical colleagues.

Which reminds me of a silly story.

A physician, a psychiatrist, a surgeon and a pathologist went duck shooting sharing one gun. The physician took the gun first and as a duck flew up he contemplated the bird carefully.

"Certainly it has a duck's beak - and, in my opinion, those feathers are definitely duck's feathers," by which time the bird was out of sight.

The psychiatrist was next and took aim as a duck flew by:-

"That's definitely a duck - but does it really feel like a duck - deep down," and the bird was out of range.

The surgeon seized the gun, took aim and shot the next bird to come into view. As it fell he turned to the pathologist.

"Tell me, old man - was that a duck?"

Now physicians can trace their speciality back over thousands of years to their origins in Egypt, Persia and Afghanistan, while the 'Johnny come lately' surgeons have only a couple of hundred years of history since they separated from the Barber - Surgeon Guild leaving the barbers to do the shaving while the surgeons did the cutting.

Psychiatrists and pathologists are really the new kids on the medical block, with barely a century of specialisation. Both rapidly established themselves as influential voices in our courts of law. Their evidence and opinions can send folk to prison or set them free. However when we were students these two newcomers were just feeling their strength but lacked the teaching base to carry us along with them. The pathologists had made a start and were supported by well written text books - their real problem was coping with over a hundred students at a time in a situation where each student needed a good close up view of the proceedings.

In order to teach their subject the Pathology Department had proudly unveiled a steeply sloped theatre to accommodate the students, with a stage down below occupied by the post-mortem table. The whole thing resembled a National Geographic reconstruction of an Aztec temple dedicated to human sacrifice.

While assistants crunched their way through the rib cage with a pair of pruning shears or circumnavigated the skull with a small saw, a tutor would recite the background clinical history like an ancient incantation. However when the offending organ that caused the death was isolated, no one could see the thing. (Today closed circuit television will have solved this). The whole performance was further animated by the ritual weighing of each organ as it was removed. The assistant would flop a liver on the scales, much like your friendly family butcher. I waited in vain to hear him say -

"Now here's a tender piece Missus - and only two bob a pound."

It was a bit bizarre and not very informative.

The Pathology Museum was even less enlightening. It was a cross between a Chamber of Horrors and Ye Olde Curiosity Shoppe. Rows of shelves marshalled sealed jars full of murky fluid and discoloured bits of people. Below the seried shelves were large cabinets containing various guns, knives and blood stained axes, involved in infamous New Zealand murders. Each item was accompanied by an uninformative label that bore the inscription 'Rex V. Smith or Rex V. Jones'.

I fondly recall one overseas student who was very impressed by these labels and was heard to remark -

"This fellow Rex got away with a lot!"

I have often wondered if the perennial shortage of pathologists that still plagues this country can be traced to the real difficulties experienced in teaching the subject.

WHAT'S IN A NAME

Sudden infant death exercised the minds of pathologists during our student days just as it does today. Up to the turn of the century its cause was well understood - it was confidently attributed to the common practice of the time, especially during winter, of having the babe in bed with the parents. In the event of sudden death it was presumed that one of the adults had inadvertently rolled onto the infant smothering it. Such deaths were written up as 'overlying' leaving both parents saturated with guilt because often neither the father nor the mother could be sure who was responsible if the child had lain between them.

As postmortem examinations on these cases became more common some enterprising pathologist noted that the thymus glands - a vague organ said to resemble the shape of the leaf of the herb thyme and found immediately beneath the breast bone, was unduly enlarged in these cases. They graced the condition with an elaborate name, 'Status Tymo-lymphaticus'. With a name like that the parents were now relieved of direct responsibility and the previous burden of guilt was lifted from the hearts of the grieving couple. For some years the world breathed easier. True, the underlying cause of the enlarged thymus remained elusive but with the discovery of agents called viruses, the profession took shelter under the implication that these minuscule pathogens would eventually prove to be the culprits.

Parents could live with 'Status Thymo-lymphaticus'. It had the Latin ring of authority endorsed by its complex spelling and tricky pronunciation. However, doubt slowly grew in the minds of some pathologists as the nature and significance of the gland was explored further. The thymus gland, they discovered, was relatively large during foetal life and could continue to grow further during normal infant development and then shrink significantly at puberty. To find an 'enlarged' thymus in infants was not necessarily an indication of significant abnormality after all. Thus the 'diagnosis' fell into disrepute and disappeared from death certificates.

By this time houses were better insulated and better heated and family sleeping habits changed. 'Overlying' became a thing of the past and victims of this syndrome were now found dead in their cots - giving us 'cot death'. The theory that a sneaky virus (still unidentified) could be responsible remained in vogue and the distraught parents were able to accept the tragedy as something beyond their control.

In the past couple of decades the public have called for a better understanding of this tragic loss of infant life and the response from both the scientific community and non scientific types has been exhaustive, commendable, and confusing. The term 'cot death' was deemed to be too inconsequential and too vague for these enlightened times, so we called for a new name that would fit in with modern marketing and campaigning. To this end we sought an appropriate acronym and came up with S.I.D.S. - 'Sudden Infant Death Syndrome'.

As everyone knows, a syndrome is a mixture of associated symptoms or causes. In this case there are no recognised symptoms - the death is too sudden for them to be identified - and there are too many hotly debated causes. The problem is that each factor attributed as a related cause imposes suggestions of negligence on the parents - particularly the mother. We have changed the name, restored the guilt, but haven't solved the problem.

IT'S IN THE BLOOD

The study of pathology naturally presupposes a knowledge of the normal before the presence and nature of the abnormal can be appreciated. To this end, as part of our First Professional studies, we were expected to be familiar with the normal limits of human blood and at the same time master the basic techniques used to prepare such material for analysis.

We were taught how to prick our thumbs with a sliver of glass and create blood smears on microscope slides as a basic step in understanding the human blood picture. Coming face to face for the first time with one's own blood, as seen through a microscope, was a strange business. Would the red corpuscles be up to scratch? Would the white cells prove to be all they should be? The presumption was that they would - given a normal state of health. It was very intimate.

Poorly printed coloured pictures were on hand depicting the landscape of normality, but even with these it took a giant leap of faith to conclude that the specimen before you, your very own blood, did really conform to the expected standard of normality.

A student in a class a year or so ahead of us encountered great difficulty in correlating the picture he saw in his blood with the illustrations available. He could not find the expected ratio of red cells to white cells and eventually called upon the tutor for assistance. His blood film was awash with white cells with only the occasional red cell in evidence. The tutor at first questioned the technique used to prepared the slide, but on repeating the procedure he sadly confirmed that the specimen was indeed correct and that the student was suffering from leucaemia - the first and last diagnosis that young man ever made.

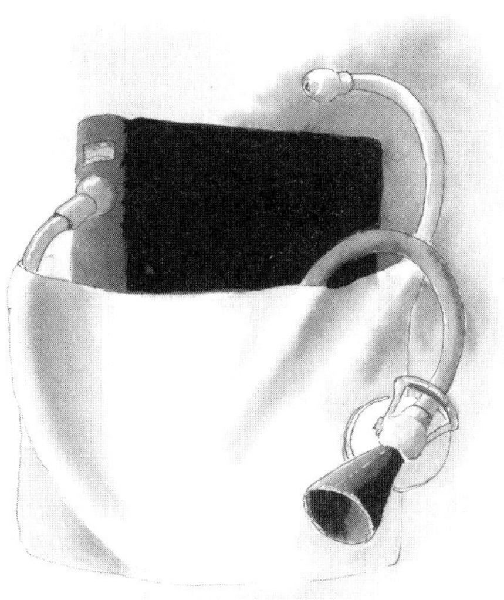

Ready to cross the road.

ON GETTING THERE

BY RULE OF THUMB

Three times each year we faced the return journey between home and university. For those who lived in the North Island this also involved an overnight passage on the Interisland Ferry that then plied between Lyttleton and Wellington. Most of us would have earned enough in the holiday to return to university by public transport, however lack of funds at the end of term reduced us to hitchhiking home.

Thus, at the end of each term thousands of students would be carried thousands of miles by generous motorists motivated simply by a desire to share - that is until motorways greatly complicated this idyllic picture.

Successful hitchhiking always was an art. The veteran carried a pack, hopefully generating an illusion of pioneering back-woods self sufficiency - an independent, self-reliant unit advancing along a predetermined course with commendable determination. The casual display of an arm extended with upraised thumb thus became less of a begging gesture and more an indication that assistance with the journey was perfectly acceptable. The kind motorist would respond through a desire to be helpful in this noble undertaking thus minimising the obvious implication of exploitation. Should your timetable be facing failure it was permissible to adopt a clearly defined limp as you doggedly pressed forward.

To merely sit on your pack by the roadside smacked of both idleness and indolence and could fail to stir the approaching driver to meritorious thoughts of generosity. Success in this venture demanded an innate understanding of the psychology involved.

Two people, trudging along together, each lumbered with a pack, presented a prospect that could exceed the generous inclinations of most drivers. The trick was to separate. One would hang about while the other walked on until safely out of sight. With the next lift secured the conversation with the driver would go something like this,

"Good heavens there's George!"

"Ya know 'im?"

"Yeh."

"'Suppose we'd better squeeze him in then."

" Hi George, fancy meeting you here."

"Yeh."

We would avoid, if possible, hitching at the very bottom of a hill. The average motorist aware of the climb ahead was more inclined to keep the revs up and pass you by. A pronounced limp has been know to overcome this problem but you could never count on it.

Hitchhikers have an unspoken obligation to instantly adapt to the political and philosophical views of their host and driver. We avoided heated debates on current affairs - they are invariably followed by awkward silences that can condense into sullenness as the miles grind past. By eagerly supporting any viewpoint one contributed to the pleasure of the journey and could rest assured that the subject would soon be dropped - preaching to the converted soon looses momentum leaving room for pleasantries and less contentious issues to ease the journey. During the '51 waterfront dispute I managed to reverse my personal opinion on this volatile, nation-wide issue, six times during a journey from Dunedin to Christchurch.

Women, however, cannot be expected to respond wholeheartedly to every moral stance that may be adopted by some male drivers. The casual suggestion, supported by body language, that they pull over and find a picnic spot must be managed with appropriate skill and cunning. The recommended reaction went something like this:-

"Well how about it - what d'ya think?"

"I guess it is ok by me, but I must warn you that I am still being treated for a very nasty disease."

This response, like a cold shower, has an established reputation for success.

Hitchhiking is not a totally selfish, one-way affair. Many company representatives engaged in a regular circuit of travel welcomed a little diversion and conversation. I recall one chap who stopped for me after a little obvious hesitation. Once in the car I was carefully interrogated about where I came from, what I did for a living and where I was bound - and all this before he was prepared to recommence his journey. After a few minutes he relaxed and apologised for the cross examination. It transpired that the last time he picked anyone up was early one morning in Invercargill and had dropped him off on the outskirts of Dunedin. Alone once again in the car he had switched on the radio to hear a chilling description of his ex passenger as an escaped prisoner. Bursting with a sense of civic responsibility he drove immediately to the Dunedin Police Station to inform them. Instead of the anticipated commendation for his responsible behaviour he was berated for involving the local constabulary in a search they had confidently predicted would not involve them. Shamefaced and humiliated he had crept away home.

On another occasion I was given an account of a similar encounter from another driver. This chap had picked up a bloke and the more they talked the more the motorist suspected that all was not well with his passenger. Eventually he made an excuse to divert briefly to a small country town supposedly to pick up some trade samples. Knowing the layout of the town he parked the car and walked around the corner to the Police Station where he described his passenger. The cop on duty was delighted and made his first arrest of the day - and probably for the month.

All new cars that entered the country in those days were individually driven from the wharf to the dealer by professional drivers who were obliged to complete the journey at a speed less than forty five miles per hour so that the engine would be 'run-in' correctly. These drivers were usually on the lookout for hitchhikers to ease their boredom. Once you adjusted to the continuous flow of speedier traffic overtaking your ride it was surprising how often you reached your destination at about the same time as everyone else. Slow but sure could win the race simply because they rarely stopped for anything more than a quick fillup with petrol.

Some rides were more memorable than others - like one ride to Taihape. About twenty miles before this rural outpost a big old Chevy responded positively to my modest signal. The driver was a diminutive Maori lad of about fifteen perched upon a cushion as an aid to better vision across the long, high bonnet of the vehicle.

As soon as I was settled in we set off at an alarming speed, surging and sliding along the narrow winding, unsealed road. The urgency of our progress was, however, adequately matched by the lad's driving skill.

"Gotta be in Taihape by two," he explained as we swung into yet another tight bend.

"Gotta meet the traffic cop and go for me license," he added reassuringly.

"Dad says we should have one in the family. We used to use me brother's but he's gone to Auckland."

At five to two we were in Taihape and as I trudged out of town my kind friend sought out his appointment with the law.

The trip from Wellington to Auckland was always the tricky bit. With luck you could make it in a day provided you took the main route through the Desert Road. Should you fail, the back-woods image became cold reality and you slept under a hedge.

Having completely run out of cash on one trip I was especially keen to make Auckland as soon as possible and was thus forced to adopt a particularly painful limp throughout the journey. It worked. By about nine p.m. my last generous driver dropped me off at the Auckland suburban bus depot.

There I stood, having successfully hitchhiked nearly five hundred miles with empty pockets and with less than ten miles to go I lacked the vital two shillings that could get me home. Confused and frustrated I limped (habit dies hard) into the public toilets and there on the floor before me lay half a crown - relief indeed!

We sat our First Professional Examinations in the middle of 1952 and I was lucky to have completed the oral examinations early, leaving a few days to spare before the end of the term and before the results would be posted under the now familiar disclaimer

"The following have failed to satisfy the examiners." Rather than hang around Dunedin waiting, I decided to hitchhike to Mount Cook and thence to Christchurch and home.

The trip to the Hermitage was quick and uneventful. I was there by early afternoon, overawed by the sheer magnitude of everything. Mountains really did tower, streams actually did rush madly along and the rocks along their shores were the size of motorcars. This was nature dressed in hyperbole.

My first task was to find a hut to shelter in overnight and with this in mind I approached an elderly chap sitting in the sun. He directed me to an old disused tramping hut upstream a little from the Heritage. Eyeing my simple pack and basic boots he gave me some thoughtful advice against wandering too far without the appropriate gear. I reassured him that I merely intended to sit at the foot of the mountains and worship them from there and would studiously avoid anything that called for the slightest vertical effort.

As I trudged of in search of my shelter and thinking about the old chap in the sun I reflected on a tale Fred Hollows had recounted the previous year. He and some friends had set off to climb Mt. Cook and during the ascent they were surprised to come upon an old fellow sitting on a rock enjoying the view. A small battered pack and an equally battered ice axe lay on the ground beside him. After the niceties of greeting had been completed they expressed both surprise and concern to find him there on the mountain side. One of the group, observing the apparent inadequacy of his equipment, hesitantly asked whether he carried crampons.

"Crampons?" he queried.

"Look I'll show you," the young climber volunteered and proceeded to demonstrate this basic climbing accessory.

"Well I never!" the old chap exclaimed, fascinated by the demonstration.

At this stage one of the party picked up the old ice axe and after examining it solemnly deposited it at the feet of his friends. Carved on the handle was "ODELL EVEREST 1924."

Odell was the first to break the embarrassed silence;

"Sorry boys - I just couldn't resist." he apologised, before commending their concern for mountain safety.

As he gathered up his pack and reclaimed the ice axe he cheerily wished them a safe journey and nimbly continued his descent.

"Good God - its just a bloody Sunday stroll to him."

As I pressed on in search of my hut I wondered vaguely if my gentle adviser could be the same climbing legend. If he was he had left his ice axe at home.

Around the corner and there it was. A sagging, rusted corrugated iron shed that encased a fireplace and two bunks. A door that still had one functioning hinge grudgingly granted entry and a glassless window, curtained with sacking, offered ventilation. With little daylight at my disposal I gathered firewood, selected the least mouldy mattress to sleep on and continued to marvel at the beauty of the place. Coffee and baked beans filled the belly and heralded sleep. The night was shared with at least two (probably more) curious restless rats.

At first light I was up and away. I had been told that a truck left the Hermitage for Pukaki at six thirty and in return for help loading it with crates of empties one could count on a ride. And so it was. The dry, dusty road back to Pukaki zig zaged first alongside the river and then the lake, playing cat and mouse with teasing glimpses of the valley, still clinging modestly to its nightdress of mist.

Pukaki at nine a.m. was deserted but at least the tiny post office was open. Here I hoped to claim a telegram sent by friends and containing my exam results. The postmistress, burdened with the expression of a school ma-am with indigestion, sullenly responded to my enquiry and pushed a brown envelope towards me as though it could contain offensive matter. Impatiently I tore it open.

"I've passed" I recklessly confided as she busily stamped very important documents.

"Oh" she sighed without missing a beat.

The bright sunny morning was now even brighter and sunnier as I took the eastern fork out of Pukaki and re-read aloud to an empty world the welcome news splattered across the yellow page.

I had trudged a couple of miles along the gently rising, unsealed road that skirted the southern shore of the lake when it dawned on me that this effort was completely unproductive. I could now see up the lake to Mt. Cook, emerging from the melting mist, right down to Pukaki village and most of the road that I had already walked. The sensible thing to do now was watch and wait. Leaving my pack by the roadside ready for instant recovery when the time came, I climbed a bank and began a very long vigil of a deserted landscape. Nothing moved, nothing at all.

I had been monarch of all I surveyed for well over an hour before the first hint of movement disturbed the scene and raised my pulse rate. In the shimmering distance a tiny dust cloud appeared and disappeared with teasing inconsistency as a vehicle snaked its way down from the Hermitage. Like slow motion in a miniature world, the tell-tale indicator crept nearer. This scenario offered three options. The vehicle could stop at Pukaki and then return, it could continue south or it could be heading for Christchurch and turn my way.

As it neared Pukaki I could identify it as a car. Apart from the morning ride this was the only moving vehicle I had seen all day and could be, the way things were going, the only one I would see. My reservation for the ferry that night could easily become a lost cause. Near Pukaki it disappeared and I was anxiously watching the south road, fearing it would take that route, when I realised in a panic it was already hurtling towards me. I scrambled down, swung on my pack and was limping along shamelessly when my long observed hope shot past without the slightest hesitation, enveloping me in a swirling dust storm.

"Bugger" erupted spontaneously.

Slowly the bitter cloud settled and there, like a mirage, stood a maroon Citroen in the middle of the road some distance ahead. Thoughtfully maintaining continuity, I limped towards it awash with relief.

The driver, a young thirty something woman was already rearranging the luggage on the back seat (fifties Citroens were not noted for boot space).

"Hi" she ventured with unmistakable American enthusiasm.

"Going far?"

"Christchurch" I replied hopefully, as I swung my pack down.

"Me too - hop in."

With my grubby load incongruously nestled among some very up market luggage I gratefully settled into the low, genuine leather bucket seat and admired the polished walnut dashboard with its incongruous central gear leaver. The long narrow bonnet flanked by the wing-like mudguards, each surmounted with a chrome headlight completed the image of tasteful luxuriance.

With the candour characteristic of her heritage she had extracted the essential elements of my life history within a matter of minutes and then spontaneously matched them with details of her own. She was on a world tour with New Zealand the last country to be visited before the return home. Upon entering each country she purchased a new Citroen, drove it everywhere and then sold it back on leaving. Her obvious wealth came from a family link with a world wide range of popular swim wear and she just loved 'Noo Ziland'.

Whenever we rushed into one of the many tight, heavily cambered bends that were a feature of the route she would exclaim as she spun the steering wheel wildly - "Don't you just *love* their low centre of gravity?" And around we would sweep without any hint of a slide. It wasn't so much the position of the centre of gravity as the front wheel drive that miraculously kept us on the road and consistently pointing in the right direction.

I had just gained enough confidence in the reliable forward tracking of the vehicle and had relaxed a little when a new danger became startlingly apparent. We were approaching an old barn with a red roof which promptly reminded her of 'back home' where, apparently, they have barns just like this one only much, much bigger. As she reminisced about her homeland and its remarkable farm buildings she moved the vehicle from the left to the right hand side of the road. Through clenched teeth I advised her that it was perhaps a little premature to anticipate her homecoming while she was still driving in a country that preferred drivers to stay left.

"Oh Gawd - I clean forgot" she sighed as we shot back to the correct side, significantly improving our chances of survival.

Clearly I now had a role to play and every time she referred to 'back home' I stood watch ready to review the rules of the road as they applied in the colonies. Slowly the road became straighter and wider and eventually we turned onto the main highway to

Christchurch. The dusty Citroen surged forwards, revelling in the smooth, straight, wide road ahead. With a stream of oncoming traffic now laying claim to the right hand side of the road my driver began to exercise her knowledge of motoring by identifying the makes of approaching cars. She could distinguish a Chevy from an Oldsmobile at half a mile. I, on the other hand, was at a disadvantage, coming from a family that had never owned a car, however it was my duty as a guest to try and join in. Eventually I recognised a Jag heading towards us and, determined to make a contribution, I observed,

"Oh look - that was a Jaguar."

Her response was both startling and dramatic. Wide eyed with alarm and distress she shouted,

"But they told me there was no snakes, tigers or other wild animals in Noo Ziland!"

I took me a while to sort out the associations and even longer to convince her that, indeed, her advisors had been correct.

As we entered the outer suburbs of Christchurch and I was confident of being on the ferry that night after all, the conversation took a new twist. She began to show an intense interest in the details of my immediate travel plans culminating in the suggestion that I simply abandon them and join her at her hotel instead.

Now here was an interesting situation. I tried to give an impression of considered deliberation while my mind rapidly sorted through the implications of the proposition. We were outside the hotel and I had my pack safely beside me on the footpath before I thanked her sincerely for the lift - it had, after all, been a very lucky journey - and virtuously strode off to join the boat train. I suppose I could have used the 'nasty disease' line but somehow it did not seem appropriate.

With many thousands of hitchhiked miles under my belt I have always felt the need to repay at least some of them. Characters weighed down by packs are a safe bet. Anyone limping is immediately suspect (but usually successful) and anyone hitching at the bottom of a hill gets a ride - together with a short opinionated lecture on the lost art of hitchhiking.

BY TRAIN

A nation that could face up to and survive the twelve hour overnight journey (second class) on the Auckland - Wellington express was a force to be reckoned with. The role that this epic journey played in preparing our armed forces for the significant part they played in the Second World War has never been adequately acknowledged. It was indeed the original survival course.

Those in the know (i.e. anyone who had done it once) prepared themselves with careful attention to detail. Arrive early at the station, empty your bladder and hire not one but two pillows. Now board the train at about its middle and claim a seat against a window about half way along the carriage. Check that the window closes completely or you will need a gas mask at each tunnel. These were the glory days of romantic steam and acrid smoke. No matter how warm the evening be prepared for a bitterly cold snap around midnight when the train passes through National Park. Extra socks, scarves and an overcoat will be appreciated in this alpine climate.

With these essential preliminaries completed it was safe to rejoin your well wishers (none of whom would have the slightest wish to accompany you), or wander along the platform to sneer at the smug first class passengers with their individual reclineable seats and first call on the heating system.

Once the hissing, huffing, tooting palaver of departure has subsided and the train is snaking through suburbia, wind your watch lest you forget to do it later and the thing fails you about lunchtime tomorrow. Now try to forget about time - Wellington is twelve hours away and the less attention paid to time the easier it will pass.

Throughout the night the journey will be punctuated with 'refreshment stops'. At these, for a modest outlay, passengers can purchase pies of indeterminate age, curiously curled sandwiches that were fresh the day before, appropriately labelled rock cakes and tannin enriched tea served in the famous railway cup. Three times the thickness of normal domestic ware these vessels were made from indestructible ceramic material that eventually would be used for heat resistant nose cones on NASA rockets. These cups were so heavy and ungainly that even students, setting up a flat, would decline them as souvenirs.

During the ski season National Park Station was a busy destination and the train would be packed with expectant skiers, many of them chattering with posh private-school accents. Each time I passed through this mecca of winter sports I was reminded of an incident involving a very down-to-earth friend who spent his holidays culling deer for the government. On this occasion he had emerged from the bush after a month, cashed his cheque and invested in a brand new, up-market pack into which he had stuffed four weeks of very dirty washing.

He was only half awake when the dimly lit train jerked and sighed to a stop and a gabble of ski enthusiasts spilled onto the station platform enveloped in an inky, ice-cold night. The train was hurtling along again before Ken fumbled in his pack for a pair of gloves and discovered the contents of his brand new acquisition had been magically transformed into a load of crisp, frilly, fragrant ladies wear.

She would probably have reached the then fashionable Chateau before discovering that she was doomed to spend a week end with a pack full of Ken's very dirty washing.

As the train descends towards sea level and dawn sneaks up, sleep depravation takes an ironic twist - daylight filters in, denying further rest. Grumpy, crumpled passengers punch pillows and twist about to escape the insistent, flickering promise of another day.

Throughout the night passenger numbers will have steadily diminished at each stop. Suddenly the balance will swing the other way as bright eyed, rested, energetic travellers board the train for the last quarter of the journey. Relaxed and animated they invade your space with their chatter as though to mock your bleary, somnolent presence.

Sleep, that proved so fugitive throughout the night must now be abandoned. Soon the journey will begin the serpentine, coast hugging entry into Wellington. To the right a sparkling ocean caresses the shore with long leisurely licks. Passengers on the left contemplate a flickering grey landscape of rocky cliff faces punctuated by the irregular vertical interjections of a myriad of multipurpose poles.

The train is now surging along, desperate to leave a good impression and ease the slow, swaying, jerky memories of the night. Long before the final station is reached the animated newcomers, impatient for their day in the capital, prepare to leave. Overnighters, on the other hand, stubbornly stay put, confident in the knowledge that once stopped this train will mercifully remain motionless for half a day.

For passengers with Wellington as their destination the ordeal is now over. However travellers destined for the South Island must now pay their 'visitor tax' - they must spend a full day in Wellington before continuing their journey further south.

If this hiatus, imposed on further travel, was sponsored by Wellington retailers it was hardly a business success. The resourceful student - albeit now in a state of serious sleep deficit - will survive on a couple of pies and a cup or two of coffee. The trick was to deposit your luggage in a locker at the station and seek out either a continuous screening movie theatre or a comfortable seat near a heater in the library, or both, and let the day drift by.

BY FERRY

The Wellington-Lyttleton Ferry was an institution unique to the nation. Even their major booking offices were decked out in the same decor as their vessels - blue with polished mahogany.

Having experienced a few stormy crossings one could feel acutely seasick simply by entering the office and booking a berth. The deck plan they spread before you had an uncanny resemblance to similar plans of slave ships.

Travellers with a nervous or introspective disposition were wise to avoid reading the small print on the back of the ticket. There, in several hundred microscopic words, the passenger was warned of those aspects of the journey for which the shipping company was not responsible. These included acts of God - piracy - war - shipwreck - collisions at sea and all circumstances that might eventuate therefrom, thereto and thereby. The sobering document suddenly became terribly relevant some years later when the "Wahine" ran aground in a storm while trying to enter Wellington Harbour, with tragic loss of life.

Impatient to escape our detention in Wellington we would wearily wander towards the ferry wharf while inner city workers thronged the pavements, packed the buses and trains and hurtled homewards leaving behind a silent city.

After six p.m. Passengers could board the ferry, claim their allotted space and casually leaning on the ship's life rails watch the ritual of preparation that animated the scene below.

Mail bags, stuffed with correspondence destined for southern readers would be loaded onto vast rope nets, their corners gathered together and swung aboard to disappear into the gaping hold. Late comers would urgently exchange abbreviated gestures of farewell with friends, family and lovers and hurry up the gangway beneath our indifferent gaze.

Suddenly the flurry of preparation would evaporate leaving a stillness like the calm that precedes the storm. The gangway - our umbilical link with the shore - would swing away. Mooring lines would splash and be hastily retrieved while the wharf slid back abandoning us to the sea.

Defying the wind chill, first timers would pace the decks and watch the city lights romantically retreat. Old hands sought out the state room for free coffee and biscuits before retiring to the economy class four and six berth cabins. Survivors of the overnight train were now at an advantage. Within minutes they would be asleep long before the ship's bows responded to the first lifting swells of the Cook Strait.

With all of New Zealand's pubs officially closed at six p.m. the ship's bar would open for trade the moment the vessel passed the three mile off shore limit. The novelty of legally imbibing alcohol during the hours of darkness was irresistible to many who would later pay for their enthusiasm with accentuated seasickness.

Most students kept clear of this novel institution. The grog was expensive and your continued supply depended directly on the generosity you lavished through tips to the serving stewards. Cynics estimated that the shipping company probably made more profit from the bar than they did through the sale of passenger tickets.

With daylight came the ritual of the morning tea round. The cabin door would suddenly burst open and a couple of indecently enthusiastic stewards, towing a jingling tea trolley, would crowd into the tiny space between the tiered bunks. By completely filling the cabin's available space they dominated the scene as they dispensed cups, two thirds filled with cool milky tea accompanied by two biscuits.

"Sugar in the top bunk sir? Berthing in ten minutes!"

Their ploy was to panic everyone into a flurry of activity and vacate the cabin ready for them to prepare for the return journey. Old hands knew better. The Ferry never touched a wharf before seven a.m.. To do so would expose the shipping company to twice the wharfage fees. We were on safe ground and took our time.

One by one the cabin's occupants would attend to the obligatory morning ablutions in the one wash basin that a few hours before had received more than its fair share of tributes to seasickness. With only room for one at a time to wash dress and pack, a little self-indulgent lie-in was in order.

At one minute to seven the veterans would appear on deck near the Purser's Office and at one second past seven the vessel would gently nudge the wharf. The crossing was completed.

The boat train that would take us to Christchurch stood alongside the ferry giving seasoned travellers another opportunity for one-up-manship. The carriage seats would all be facing one way. Veterans would flip their seat back over into the opposite mode before settling in. They knew that the train would eventually move off in the opposite direction leaving the new chums confused and facing backwards. It was these little touches that separated the men from the boys.

With Christchurch came the chance for breakfast. Opposite the Christchurch Railway Station there was an eatery called "The Hole in the Wall". This modest establishment served cooked flounder that completely over hung the plate. With one of these aboard survival for the journey south was assured.

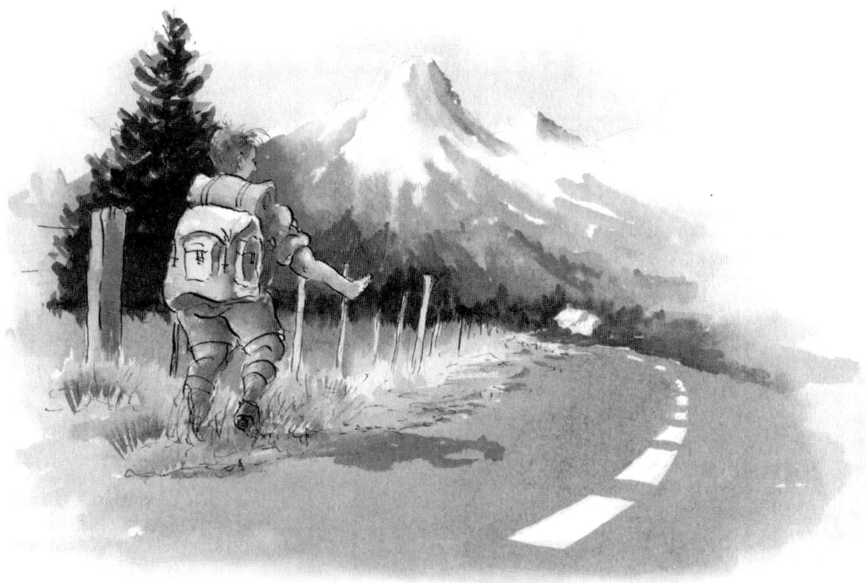

Thumb power.

DRUGS OF CHOICE AND OTHER DIVERSIONS

Tea, in the early fifties, was the cup that cheered and the nation's chief source of caffeine. In this regard we mirrored the preferred beverage of the old Empire and the modern Commonwealth which produced it. The sociable sipping of tea gently encouraged conversation and punctuated the day with little oases of calm and recreation. 'Tea and sympathy' was enough for our parents recovering from a depression followed by a world war but their children, seeking more fire in their bellies and more caffeine in their veins, were turning to coffee.

Some tea rooms moved upmarket to become cafes and a few New Zealand homes could even rustle up a percolator for special occasions. Flickering images on countless movie screens portrayed private detectives, newspaper reporters and their editors all in hot pursuit of truth and justice, buoyed up in their worthy endeavours by regular bursts of caffeine.

Here was a beverage that could extend the day's work well into the night and clear a hangover next morning with one hot strong black cup. The role of pharmacology in supporting a life style was becoming established and with the marketing of instant coffee, instant gratification was at hand.

Five hundred years ago, in the burnt out ends of the fifteenth century, Christopher Columbus found the Indians of South America ritually smoking tobacco leaf in their 'pipes of peace' Fifty years later the drug was established in Europe, still associated with the dubious image of peace and tranquillity. By the 1950's tobacco consumption in the Western World had reached its popular peak.

Throughout the two world wars that clouded the first half of the twentieth century governments on both sides ensured a steady supply of the tranquillising leaf for their troops. By now tobacco was cheap and eminently taxable but smoking it was still restricted to males by four centuries of social convention. The female half of all populations were essentially non smokers. After a meal the ladies withdrew to the withdrawing room while their partners sat around the table sipping port and smoking tobacco.

It was the Second World War that changed all that. While the 'bread winners' were overseas women temporarily replaced them in the factories and in taking over this traditional male role they adopted two previously male characteristics - they wore trousers and smoked cigarettes. Come the peace they quietly returned to the kitchen taking their new dress code and a taste for tobacco with them, heralding the first murmurings of a renewed campaign for sexual equality.

About seventy per cent of the adult population now smoked tobacco - and that included students, nurses and the medical profession in general. Tobacco had replaced religion as the 'opium of the people'. Every public waiting area was liberally supplied with ash trays, including doctor's waiting rooms and the bedside lockers of hospital patients. I well remember a Chest Physician who chain smoked through every consultation and eventually died of lung cancer.

The world's nicotine-stained tranquillity was rudely disturbed in 1953 when Britain's Minister of Health suddenly announced that there was a 'strong presumption' that tobacco smoking was linked with the incidence of lung cancer. Smoking doctors were quick to question the validity of this claim but already the tide was turning. Today, nearly half a century later, the profession aims to be 'smoke free'.

Two years after the 'strong presumption' warning the pharmaceutical industry launched its first synthetic tranquilliser promising a new source of inner peace and a whole new raft of health threatening complications.

Most smokers and many non smokers chose alcohol as their preferred recreational drug. Labourers and students could afford beer and as most students worked in labouring jobs for part of each year this choice implied a comfortable sharing. The manual workers would stick faithfully to their choice but successful students could eventually graduate to the top shelf - and most did.

In the fifties the right to consume alcohol beyond one's place of residence was not only governed by age (over 21) it was also strictly regulated by time of day and day of the week. Pubs, the only legal servers of alcoholic beverages to the general public, were obliged to cease service at six p.m., discharge their patrons into the street and close their doors. On the Sabbath they remained closed all day.

Guests, booked into an hotel however, were especially blessed. They could drink at the House Bar for as long as mine host cared to keep the bar open. Thus a citizen who faced arrest for 'being found on licensed premises after hours' was magically transformed into a legal drinker by the mere possession of a room key.

Without exception every pub would obediently cease to serve alcohol to the general public at six each evening. However most would open their back doors about an hour later to engage in a brisk, though illegal, afterhour trade.

The system was simple. A thirsty citizen, having solemnly knocked three times at the pub's back door, would be surveyed briefly through a side window and on approval, be admitted to a dimly lit bar further darkened by an overhanging haze of tobacco smoke, where alcohol at inflated prices was served in a whisper.

Each entrant would be greeted by a sudden hush in the carefully modulated conversation while fellow law breakers took stock of the new arrival. Any stranger, recognised as such by the regulars, would be informed of the optimum escape route in the event of a raid before the assembled company could relax and take up conversation once more.

The tense atmosphere recalled scenes from old war-time escape movies and generated an adrenaline lift that combined strangely with the alcohol ingested. You could pay good money to watch exciting films - here you paid good money to take part.

The police, for their part, made every effort to be fair, sharing their attention evenly over the pubs in their district. Having been raided, a publican could reasonably conclude that the next two weeks or so would be peaceful.

In the event of an unwelcome visit the pub concerned would quickly notify neighbouring establishments by coded telephone messages. On receipt of such information the neighbour would quickly empty its patrons into the backyard where they would be staring skywards with contrived innocent concentration when the investigating officers arrived. It was as though pub backyards had suddenly become the common meeting place for local astronomy clubs.

Eventually, as the police withdrew through the front door, the thirsty patrons would re-enter via the back and the evening would resume as though nothing had happened. Even their half empty glasses would be where they left them prior to evacuation.

Students rarely drank in pubs after hours - a decision based more on the added expense involved than on any innate respect for the law. Instead we reserved episodes of alcoholic excess for the celebration of life's milestones including the completion of exams. Because less than one student in a hundred owned a car and even fewer could afford taxis the prudent celebrant only attended parties within walking distance of their residences.

Beer for a student bash was usually purchased directly from the breweries in five gallon kegs. Medical students tended to support Speights Brewery because a member of this prestigious family held an important post in the Department of Surgery. We hoped that such brand loyalty might somehow be acknowledged in favourable examination results at a later date.

Music was the second important ingredient for a party and mercifully the fifty's gramophone lacked significant amplifier output. Thus music could only be played at normal volume before gross distortion intervened. The great novelty of the times was the vinyl long playing record which was steadily replacing the brittle 78's. On the eve of a party the residents would go to great lengths to hide away their precious records leaving out only those that they were prepared to offer up as possible sacrifices.

Inevitably, as the night wore on, liquor supplies would diminish although demand was still manifest. This was where Dunedin's illegal emergency home delivery service clicked in. The necessary funds would be gathered through individual contribution and a shopping list drawn up. This order would then be telephoned to the nearest taxi office, they, in turn, would relay the order to the local pub and send a cab around to collect it. The driver would then deliver the goods collecting payment for the grog plus the taxi fare. Convenient, practical and illegal.

In those days a joint of cannabis was known as a 'reefer' and was smoked occasionally by visiting merchant seamen ashore from the South American run. Local interest in the drug was limited to some musicians (particularly drummers) who believed that it enhanced their performance on stage - and to expressionist painters who found it inspirational. Students in general stayed with accessible, predictable alcohol.

We were probably the last generation of students to settle for the trilogy of tea, tobacco and alcohol to smooth out the passage of time.

ENTERTAINMENT AND LEISURE

In the fifties New Zealand admitted one hundred and twenty students each year to its only medical school, well below the number necessary to compensate for retirements and current population growth. The books were balanced in part by importing medical graduates from overseas, especially from Britain and South Africa. At this time, ironically, the number of New Zealand doctors working overseas exceeded the number working in their homeland.

In the immediate post war years competition for a seat in the school was extremely intense. Understandably, places were first reserved for all those returned service personnel who had passed the entrance examination (Medical Intermediate) and a further four seats were held for similarly qualified Maori students.

When these commitments had been met the remaining seats were fiercely competed for by several hundred applicants. Allocation was made on the basis of overall academic achievement and many students spent an extra year or more in further study in order to move up the waiting list.

However, once a place in the school had been secured, interpersonal battles were largely over and each student enjoyed the same opportunity to emerge at the other end with the necessary documents that would empower them to practice medicine in New Zealand and a good part of the world.

We were now engaged in a common task and there was a novel willingness to share knowledge and experiences. Furthermore, because we all followed the same timetable and completed exams at the same time, we would become a compact academic and social unit that would not only remain intact for the next four years but would eventually celebrate reunions from time to time for the rest of our lives.

Periodically, during our study years, someone would organise a function aptly described as a 'class bash' - 'bash' being the operative word. A successful bash arose like spontaneous combustion, from the conjugation of an alcohol supply, a dance band and a venue. The first two were easily arranged but the event's location was always a problem because in any year other student groups would also punctuate periods of study with episodes of celebration, leaving residual images of mayhem in the collective memory of venue managers. The trick was to find an establishment 'under new management' and home in on the tenderfoot innocents.

The success of a class bash was measured by the degree of amnesia generated by the event. Thus, by definition, a poorly remembered occasion must have been a noteworthy celebration.

While our younger siblings prepared to gyrate to the sinister temptations of Rock and Roll we clung to the safer rhythms of Swing and Jazz and, comfortably coupled for dancing, glided to the sophisticated lilt of the waltz, fox-trot and quick step, between drinks. Most dance bands played without amplification, making us the last generation to enjoy social interchange without the risk of significant hearing loss.

In this strictly regulated environment a partner was a prerequisite, and where male students outnumbered female by ten to one it was necessary to look beyond the institution to find a companion. The Schools of Physiotherapy and Home Science plus the ever hospitable Nurses' Home willingly restored the appropriate gender balance

Otago University, with its abundance of specialist schools, staged more academic balls than any other tertiary institution in the country. These episodes of implied tutor-student goodwill were scatted through the dark, cold, winter months with exhausting regularity.

Balls were to class bashes as maypole dances are to riots. They were expensive affairs, especially for the male student who was expected not only to fund the 'double ticket' and hire an evening suit but to purchase a corsage for his lady as well. This petite floral tribute, destined to adorn his partner's dress, cost about a weeks rent and rarely survived uncrushed beyond the supper waltz. It was the thought that counted of course, but the cost/benefit ratio was always dubious.

Male accessories for the evening usually included a silver or gold cigarette case (Russian on one side and Turkish on the other) together with a matching cigarette lighter. The case would be flipped open in a generous sharing gesture at every opportunity. Even non smoking men were often so armed, thus expressing tolerance and a plea for inclusion.

Catering for balls rarely extended to the provision of alcohol - an omission that many felt obliged to correct at a personal level. A reasonable supply of spirits (usually whisky) could be secreted about one's person in a hip flask. This flattened, slightly concave, screw capped, silver bottle was designed to slip into a hip or inside jacket pocket while still retaining an acceptable impression of sartorial elegance. Today, like snuff boxes, they are collector's items but in mid century they simply anticipated today's B.Y.O..

Lucky indeed was the young lady whose partner had access to a car. Few students could afford taxi fares so the prudent male carefully sought a partner who lived within high heeled walking distance of the venue. Fortunately Dunedin was a compact city with a centrally placed Nurse's Home.

The wireless (radio) and picture theatre (cinema) offered passive entertainment. The former, comfortably aglow with valves and ironically festooned with wires, was free, while the latter, usually in glorious black and white, was affordable to all.

From the radio emerged a comforting clutter of soppy soaps, silly quizzes and incredibly boring request sessions in which the time taken to read out the names and locations of the requesters usually vastly exceeded the time taken to play the item. After each playing the announcer would identify the appropriate recording company with the solemn observation. "That was a Decca recording".

Within this bland sea of sound the B.B.C. flashed intermittently like a beacon offering our basic menu of overseas news. If an event was not newsworthy in London it was unlikely to become news in New Zealand. Thus 'Mother England' helped us retain the comforting insularity of the time.

However a B.B.C. Broadcasting bonus came in the form of a comedy series written by Frank Muir and Denis Nordon called "Take it from Here". A prophetic title because it generally challenged the pedantic censorship boundaries that prevailed, opening the way for "The Goon Show" and eventually "Monty Python" on television.

The authors cleverly wove innuendo and double entendre through their work with liberating effect. A typical example involved an outdoors scene and included dialogue which went something like this:- "Oh Mavis, its so quiet here - just you, me, and that couple over there on the verge." What sanctimonious arbiter of public morals could challenge that item without revealing that they saw sexual content where none need exist? Cinema offered episodic escape. Hollywood, responding to the challenge of T.V. in U.S.A. produced spectacles like "The Robe" and "Greatest Show on Earth" while still producing less expensive classics such as "High Noon" and "African Queen". All were made within the stifling 'Hollywood Code' of self-censorship soon to be challenged by "A Streetcar Named Desire".

In New Zealand, television's challenge to cinemas was still decades away leaving our city picture theatres comfortably filled for four sessions each day (except of course on Sunday). Some theatres still carried signs that promised their patrons "talkies".

By now the post-war British film industry was at its peak releasing a string of very successful features that included "The Third Man", "The Lavender Hill Mob" and "The Man in the White Suit" - (one of our year gained brief casual employment by parading around in a white suit to promote this film).

Film distribution in New Zealand was a conservative though profitable affair. Very few prints of a new production would enter the country and they would be exhibited first in the main centres until patronage began to contract. The reels, packed in aluminium boxes, would then be delivered, usually by train, to their suburbs and thence to lesser towns and eventually their suburbs. Finally, a year or two later, the print, patched with hundreds of splices would jump and splutter in remote country halls where patrons often sat on their saddles rather than leave them on their horses patiently waiting outside. Thus the nation's exposure to other (selected) cultures was completed and the entire population appropriately entertained.

Recorded music was in a state of flux. The heavy, brittle 78 r.p.m. records, with their limited playing time were now being replaced by the technologically superior, light weight vinyl long playing discs. These in their turn, demanded a new turn table and amplifier surrounded by state of the art speakers. High fidelity was born - pushing recorded music into a luxury bracket beyond the reach of most students. The revolutionary transistor had been perfected in 1948 but existing contracts for valve manufacture would delay, for about twenty years, their eventual dominating role.

Bing Crosby and Frank Sinatra had introduced a hesitant world to Swing but for us Jazz still ruled and Louis Armstrong was king. Meanwhile folk younger than us were soon to be seduced by the hypnotic beat of Rock and Roll.

Musicians were scattered through the student body and from time to time a few would come together for a 'jam' session. One of our year played a mean slap base, so much so that soon after graduation he moved to U.S.A. surrendering medicine for a career in music. Before he left New Zealand, Lyn Christie taught me a haunting jazz version of "The Three Bears" which I adapted and later crooned gently to children while I anaesthetised them.

Capping week, the highlight of the acaedemic year, was characterised by an incongruous blend of ceremony and epic overindulgence. Graduates from the previous year would assemble in May, deck themselves in hired academic robes and formally parade through the city's streets before taking their place in the colourful, ancient ritual of capping. In the evening, dressed in their finest they would converge on the Town Hall to enjoy the Graduation Ball.

Each year, as part of the capping celebrations, those students with a special interest in theatre produced the 'Students' Review' - a stage show where current political and social issues would be aired with scant regard for the laws of libel. Here macho men would shamelessly cross-dress as ballet dancers and perform exerts from "Swan Lake" with the finesse and delicacy commonly associated with a rugby scrum.

This was the one time each year that the University reached out to Dunedin's citizens and entertained them. Eventually this bridge would collapse as the University grew and the pressure on the individual student intensified, leaving neither time nor energy to sustain the link.

Undergraduates, capitalising on the relaxed, forgiving atmosphere of Capping Week would support the Capping procession by dressing outrageously and parading through the city on a series of floats festooned with satirical posters. From this vantage point they would attack the public with waterpistols in one hand and a collection box in the other. The worthy nature of the charity being supported served as a handy license for exaggerated behaviour.

The 'good cause' scheduled to benefit from my first experience of a student procession was the new and then little known Intellectually Handicapped Children's Society. The much older Crippled Childrens' Society was well supported by the public. This organisation was dedicated to the needs of children suffering from diseases of bones, muscles and joints but its policy excluded children with intellectual problems.

I.H.C. was the new kid on the block. Their organisers assured us that the number of children suffering intellectual handicap was increasing steadily. The question was why - and the answer was penicillin. There had always been a percentage of babes born with such handicaps but many of these died of pneumonia at a young age. Thanks to penicillin more and more of these children were now surviving. The same antibiotics that spared the lives of intellectually disabled children were also preventing the crippling effects of bone and joint disease in older children. Mercifully a combination of immunisation and antibiotics would soon erode the ranks of crippled children and change the face of children's charities for the rest of the century.

SEX AND CELIBACY

"The virgins' retreat," was an unkind aphorism frequently applied to Nurses' Homes by self deluded, macho male students when bragging amongst themselves. The disdain implied in this observation would evaporate immediately accounts of their mythical conquests were challenged. Most students of both sexes, in those days, *were* virgins – though few would admit it.

Student marriage was extremely rare and living in sin was simply not an option. However, like a victory parade after years of wartime deprivation, most students wed within a year of graduation. Celibacy the impostor – triumphantly overthrown.

Given the state of contraception at that time and irrespective of moral considerations, sexual abstinence was a pragmatic, prudent choice. Inter-gender encounters were limited to occasional episodes of 'heavy petting' – neatly summed up by one of my peers as "up-town shopping for down-town goods" and touched on by an anatomy lecturer with the classic "those of you who study anatomy by Braille will know that the female breast ----."

The contraceptive pill, that would eventually give us mixed flatting and Woodstock, was a decade away. Most contraceptive measures were inherently unreliable and remarkably inaccessible. Spermicidal creams, jellies and fizzy, insertable tablets were about as safe as Russian Roulette, leaving the time honoured condom as the safest choice in a risky undertaking. In theory all adults had legal access to a supply of contraceptive agents, the problem was navigating the tricky waters that a cynical society carefully placed in their way.

Chemists were one of the few retailers entitled to sell contraceptive products – though they were not obliged to do so. Their stocks, hidden from sensitive public gaze, lay beneath the counter guarded religiously by a bevy of young female shop assistants.

Even tough truck drivers would hover about the shop, anxiously trying to attract the attention of the male pharmacist so that they could indicate, man to man, the nature of the intended transaction. If, however, our driver had inadvertently chosen a shop under catholic management there would be no purchase. A little street savvy was essential.

A service of doubtful legality that every truck driver appreciated, was offered by men's hairdressers. At the completion of the trim and just after the offer of three drops of Bay Rum to the scalp your considerate barber might whisper, "need anything for the weekend sir?"

An affirmative nod would see a small discrete packet appear along with your change. Little wonder that haircuts at two weekly intervals were popular with men in those days.

Should you anticipate 'weekend needs' between trims you could attend the retail half of the barber shop. Here you would place your hand flat on the counter with a half crown coin gripped between middle and fore finger while nonchalantly pretending an interest in a jar of Brylcream. This nationally understood signal would be answered with the appropriate wee half crown packet. Had you, unknowingly, chosen to patronize a catholic barber you could always settle for the Brylcream.

Tabloid newspapers and some down-market magazines frequently carried advertisements offering to supply by post 'your personal private needs delivered through the mail in a plain wrapper!' This service was especially popular in those small towns where both the chemist and the barber attended mass.

The risk of pregnancy was extremely high among actively courting couples, particularly where engagements of one or two years were commonly imposed by parents on either side. A sort of engagement without engagement. Marriage was the only socially acceptable response to any pregnancy outside wedlock and this ceremony would be organized with righteous haste and a grim determination that gave rise to the colourful term a 'shot gun wedding'. Babes born after such accelerated nuptuals often featured in the newspaper Birth Notices as 'premature', in a vain bid to confuse the calculations of nosey neighbours and unsympathetic relatives. Indeed the number of births so described greatly exceeded the official statistics for prematurity every year.

When marriage, for whatever reason, was not an option, the plight of the pregnant woman (usually a teenager) was especially miserable. Instead of being a bride at the centre of adulation and public good wishes she would find herself shamed as an 'unmarried mother-to-be' and secretly packed away for a long, lonely holiday 'up north' where she would face, among strangers, her confinement, delivery and the immediate adoption of her babe to an anonymous couple.

The Maori community, on the other hand, rarely treated 'unmarried mothers' in this insensitive way. Instead, they gave the continuing support of their families and if adoption was to be undertaken it would usually be an 'open' one within the family.

The extramarital pregnancy that did not lend itself to shot guns or sudden holidays abroad could be dealt with by abortion, either legal or illegal. The 'legal' option was so narrowly defined in law that very few cases qualified. Two senior medical consultants had to agree, among other things, that the continuation of the pregnancy would most certainly lead to the death or permanent disability of the mother or would plunge her into a state of permanent mental illness. Women suffering from advanced tuberculosis or gross rheumatic heart disease might qualify but all those encumbered with lesser burdens would be declined.

A more subtle approach was sometimes available to well-to-do middle class folk who could find their way to a sympathetic gynaecologist with a private consultant practice and access to private operating facilities. The specialist would adopt the view that the case was simply one of irregular periods (confirmed by his clinical notes) and should benefit from a good clean out of the uterus, and the sooner the better. Later, the advent of reliable pregnancy testing made it very difficult to sustain this convoluted rationalisation.

The third avenue led straight to the back street abortionist who literally operated from back street slum accommodation, away from public gaze. Some were males but a remarkable number were women who claimed at least some nursing or midwifery experience. Their fee, to be paid in cash, was around fifty pounds – which in those days amounted to about ten weeks wages for a labourer.

This was a city service that reached out to the public through hotel bars and some taxi drivers. The father to be, burdened with guilt, often undertook to research the market and try to find the fee. It was his partner, however, who faced serious threats to her life, future health and fertility without understanding the risk involved. The abortionist, on the other hand, clearly understood the potential consequences of the undertaking and took elaborate precautions to avoid incrimination.

The pregnant woman faced a trinity of potentially fatal complications. She risked death from massive haemorrhage, overwhelming infection or from shock. Haemorrhage and infection usually took some hours or days to develop, long after she had left the premises. Death through shock tended to be immediate and caused abortionists the most concern, leaving them with a body on their hands.

The terrible trinity of complications are all avoidable, given appropriate surgical practice. Shock is prevented by anaesthesia, infection by adequate sterilization of equipment while haemorrhage is reduced by drugs and is correctable by appropriate transfusion.

Because the back street abortionist practiced illegally we have no statistics covering either their numbers or their activities. Some grim evidence of their operations did appear fairly regularly in all public hospitals. Woman, deathly pale from haemorrhage and/or pelvic infection would be admitted as acute emergencies, insisting, even with their dying breath, that they had not been recently pregnant. They all knew that they had colluded in an illegal act and shared guilt with their abortionist who thus remained shielded by their denial. Mercifully by then we had the antibiotics and transfusion technology to save most of them. We could not, however, heal the mental trauma, nor could we restore the fertility that was usually lost as a result of gross pelvic infection.

Abortion on demand is as old as the hills and no doubt will continue to be the subject of future debate, led mainly by those who are unlikely to ever become pregnant. At least our back streets are finally free of the desperate consultations that once resulted in so much misery and death. The social pressure that once refused to accept any birth outside marriage must carry a share of this back street shame.

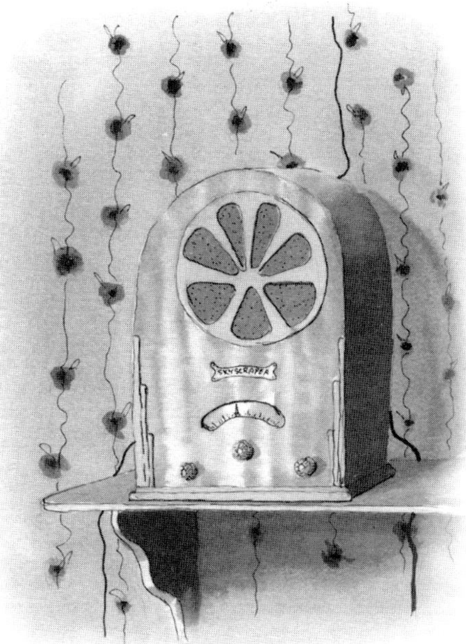

Wireless.

THE MEEK SHALL INHERIT

There can be no doubt that the fifties was a great decade for students. Unemployment figures then averaged thirty eight each month and the department knew each of them by their given names. Almost every factory had a notice out front offering work. Imports were heavily restricted to protect local manufacturers and the choice of goods in our shops was very limited - but one's capacity to buy was protected by full employment.

The first Labour government had put in place a scheme by which children of working class families could aspire to tertiary education through a system of examinations supported by a declaration of parental income. A living allowance was included to support those of us who had to live away from home. In return the successful applicant could be required to work for two years at the direction of the state. (Medical services to the Chatham Islands were usually maintained in this way.) Should a student fail and have to repeat a year of study, support would be withheld during that period - a very effective incentive.

With work freely available it was a simple matter to lift the bank balance each holiday and most of us soon had a relationship with an employer that ensured continuity of employment opportunities. Well paid casual work was often advertised in the extensive 'Situations Vacant' columns of the newspapers. One worth watching for always began "Brush hands wanted." This plea came from a firm that specialised in painting anti-fouling on the bottom of ships.

I responded to this once and found myself, along with a hundred or so others, standing in a courtyard down by the city wharves in Auckland. A chap with a clipboard was moving solemnly among us appraising each hopeful with a cold calculating eye. It reminded me of accounts of the slave markets of yesteryear. However he sensibly refrained from pinching our biceps before entering our names on his list.

Eventually the hundred would-be hands were selected, recorded and directed to the 'launch steps' by the harbour Ferry Terminal where two passenger launches, with motors idling in anticipation, awaited us.

During the journey across the harbour I noticed that some of my fellows carried rolled up sugar bags and I briefly speculated on their possible intentions. Nearing our destination the experienced hands carefully surveyed the skyline and confidently announced that the dock was empty. The intended object of our attention, a freighter, was still making its approach. This knowing observation confirmed that the job would easily last two days.

And so it was. It was well after lunch before the ship had entered the giant swimming pool of a dock and the watertight doors had closed behind it. Once the vessel was moored in position and pumping out had begun we climbed onto pontoons tethered to the ship's side. Armed with scrapers that looked like heavy duty garden push-hoes we chipped and scraped away at the abundant marine growth that had accumulated just below the waterline. Meanwhile the pumps struggled on as the dock emptied.

The moment the ship's keel settled on the raised central ridge that ran the length of the dock we were ordered out while the ship was braced in position. Enormous wooden struts, like giant power poles, were jammed between the vessel's sides and the terraced wall of the dock opposite, thus propping her on an even keel while the water drained away.

While most of us stood around supervising the procedure, (after all we had a vested interest in the stability of the vessel) some of our number migrated towards the pumping station where the last of the water awaited expulsion. Suddenly this remnant pool burst into boiling activity and my sugar sack-carrying mates dashed down to claim their share of the trapped fish now flapping helplessly on the dock floor. The day was over and already some of us were assured of a fish dinner.

Next morning our vessel looked strangely out of place - like an enormous whale trapped outside its environment and braced in position by a series of poles leaving two propellers and a rudder curiously exposed to the common gaze.

Fifty of us on each side, standing on the dock floor and armed with our reinforced hoes began the arm aching, neck wracking task of scraping away the extensive marine growth from the hull above, while fishy juices ran down the handles and dripped from our elbows.

By lunchtime the much travelled fauna and flora now littered the dock floor leaving a clean, rust-pocked hull above ready for painting.

We gratefully traded our hundred hoes for fifty extension ladders, fifty paint brushes and fifty pots of paint. From here on it was a two man affair. One stood at the base of the ladder holding the side rails with feet jammed against the ladder ends to prevent the thing slipping while the trusting partner climbed up to the top and painted the first metre below the waterline. Having painted as far as you could reach you gladly descended and swapped roles. At the same time two chaps, encased in paint - stiffened overalls which included a hood with a glass visor, sprayed the rest with longhandled spray guns.

By mid afternoon the transformation was complete. She stood proudly, enhanced by her fresh coat of paint and polished propellers impatient for the return of her element. With a sense of collective contentment we wandered down to the wharf to collect our pay and join the launches for the return trip. Next time, I resolved, I would take a sugar sack.

As it transpired this would be my only experience as a 'brush hand'. I soon found work a short bikeride from home at a local brickworks and would return there regularly until graduation.

Short stints of labour were just as good for the body and soul as for the pocket. They provided the perfect escape from text books and lectures and lasted just long enough to render the inevitable return to academic life welcome once again. Mercifully, for the student, this idyllic balance between mental and physical effort would eventually end leaving our workmates to build a life around the monotony of endlessly repeated tasks. For a doctor, a special by-product of this work experience was the ease with which one could communicate in two worlds - a sort of social bilingualism. A capacity that patients often valued above other professional skills.

Working in a factory that employed a hundred or so workers was an interesting experience. The establishment was big enough to accommodate a hierarchy of skills and yet small enough to retain a sense of family into which anyone, who was a fully paid up member of the Labourer's Union, would be acceptable. Our unionman was a gentle Welshman who operated the flower pot machine and of course coached the church choir.

"Us can do with it," he would say as you paid your dues and received your membership card.

In a fifties brickworks the products were moved everywhere by a combination of manpower and a wheel barrow. The barrows were a triumph of evolved design. Their load was so arranged that when in the wheeling position the centre of gravity of the load lay directly over the axle. Once on this point of balance the operator required only slight *downward* pressure on the handles to retain equilibrium and wheel the thing around. It was a bit like riding a bike - once you had the knack you could shift loads around the place with only modest effort.

The whole place operated on a system of gangs, each dedicated to a specific task. The 'Off Bearers' wheeled soft, freshly made bricks from the brick machine and arranged them on drying racks. The air dried product was gathered by the 'Crowders' and wheeled to the kiln where the 'Setters' skilfully stacked the material before the 'Burners' fired the thing up. Once cool, the 'wicket' (a temporary door loosely built of bricks plastered with mud to seal the kiln during firing) had been removed, and the 'Draggers' moved in to transport the fired contents to the stack outside, ready for sale. The whole place resembled an ant's nest with teams in double lines moving outwards and then returning along the same route as items were moved around.

Wages were satisfactory, the owners made their profit yet the product could only be afforded by the well-to-do. Brick houses were not for everyman. In a way this was a cost against full employment. With automation, bricks would be cheaper, profits would be higher and jobs harder to find.

The first hint of mechanisation in our factory came with the purchase of a front-end loader to transport coal from the stack outside and deposit it around the kilns. (A job that nobody liked). Non the less this new acquisition was viewed with suspicion by many of the old hands. Management responded with commendable tact, decreeing that the only person allowed to drive the thing would be the union rep. who could thus ensure that no jobs would be lost. Our gentle Welshman drove that loader around the place with a grin from ear to ear, as though he could hear a heavenly choir faultlessly rendering

"For we, like sheep have gone astray." Like it or not the battle was already lost.

A mile or so away a neighbouring brickyard was building an automated unit to run alongside their conventional system. For a few years more jobs were available but eventually the old, labour intensive method, would become redundant. Bricks would be cheaper but Mr. Everyman (and his wife) now needed job security before they could build with them.

Apart from the prophetic front-end loader my employers resisted further automation and within a decade the site of the old works was occupied by a shopping complex and the 'Staff Wanted' notices had disappeared from every factory front as automation moved us all into the second half of the twentieth century.

But that was then and this is now and fifty years have brought some interesting reversals. The men I worked with in the brickworks were lean and fit while our bosses were overweight and short of breath. Today's bosses pay good money to stay trim by 'working out' regularly while the poor are overweight through a diet of cheap food and underactivity.

The opportunity for physical work, once the exclusive domain of the poor, is now something the middle class willingly pay to do themselves at work-outs, together with the fashionable 'working clothes' that go with it. Furthermore, having virtually lost the opportunity to work, the very existence of the poor is denied today - we have successfully hidden them under that pathetic, almost obscene euphemism, 'the lower socio-economic group' and turned them once again into an embarrassment.

Hand in hand with the newfound passion for middle class fitness came the determination to quit smoking. The stereotypes of cigar chomping, chain-smoking executives began to fade three decades ago. For centuries tobacco had remained the indulgence of the rich but this century has seen the balance swing away leaving the poor as the last resource for tobacco tax, (a cool $900,000,000 annually at last count).

ODD JOBS

All universities, mindful of the perceived wisdom of the time - namely that bright minds should be carried about the place in healthy bodies - decreed that Wednesday afternoons would be lecture-free and dedicated to the glory of sport. To make up for any lost time they also decreed that teaching would occupy each Saturday morning.

I wonder if today's temples of tertiary education still preach the mantra linking sport with health? Football, in all its varieties is already an orthopaedic surgeon's dream as damaged joints quietly moulder into osteoarthitis and will eventually be ripe for replacement. Few of today's stars will twinkle into middle age and beyond without at least one artificial joint to limp around on.

Some years ago I was asked to give the nurses a lecture on osteoarthitis and needed some x-rays that would illustrate the condition for them. I consulted one of the orthopaedic surgeons for a few names to look up in the X-ray Department. He smiled and gave me one name - that of a local All Black - and assured me that there would be enough material in that packet to lecture for a week.

We have already passed the point where continued striving to excel is beyond the player's best interests for continued good health, just as we have pushed the development of the motorcar to the point that it now performs beyond our capacity to drive the thing safely and have to add devices like air bags to compensate for some of the design features that have increased its lethal power - and euphemistically called them *safety* features. Similarly, in many sports, expectations now exceed the body's capacity to function without continued damage to its component parts. (Some competitors even call on drugs to compound the situation). Perhaps it is already time to stick health warnings on sports equipment.

My only experience of organised sport came during primary school days when, by mistake, I found myself in a bare-foot rugby team for one eminently forgettable game. Even at that tender age I had worked out that the healthiest place in a rugby match was to be wherever the ball wasn't. By studiously avoiding it I managed to complete the game remarkably clean and free of bruises. Before they could throw me out I took on a paper run that conveniently excused me from further sporting encounters. Paper runs are, after all, very good exercise - and you get paid.

Dunedin had an informal pool of health-giving casual work for Wednesday afternoons - passed from student to student like a dose of flu. Current indebtedness was the only real incentive necessary to complicate one's life in this way - and restored solvency was the signal to pass the job onto someone currently in need.

In this way I found myself gardening for three bob an hour, closely supervised by the householder, an old chap in gumboots who was still reliving his personal dream of glorious authority that had doggedly clung to him since World War One. The faithfully maintained, slightly ridiculous, handle-bar moustache told all.

He stood behind me like a second shadow as I separated weeds from more desirable herbage. As his badge of authority he gripped a short piece of bamboo which may once have supported a Christmas Lily and now tapped impatiently against the top of his right gumboot, with the rhythmic precision of a nervous tic. Only officers carried swagger sticks - only officers needed to.

After a couple of hours of threatening supervision, the tension was magically relieved by the musical tinkle of tea cups. Enter Mrs. 'Major' through french doors left, carrying a tea tray. Generously proportioned for her diminutive stature she arranged the afternoon tea things and called cheerfully, and rather incongruously, "Come along boys."

The ominous tapping stopped after one conclusive slap - my signal to 'jump to'. Obediently he led me to the repast. The stick of authority was put aside on an empty chair - signalling a period of informality. While I enjoyed the fresh scones and strawberry jam his gracious wife, with blue eyes a-twinkle, maintained a polite yet interested conversation.

Suddenly I felt sorry for her - trapped with this man who was in turn a prisoner of his own past. His most articulate response was a grunt, yet she chatted on with genuine curiosity and honest compassion. She reminded me of a cage bird let out to sing.

With a frown he consulted his watch, a-dangle on its gold chain and with a grunt of resignation reached for his stick as he arose. Conversation ceased with startling abruptness. The tea things were obediently gathered and the cage door closed.

After this interval, act one was repeated. Eventually I had served my time and was allowed to retreat, enriched with my earnings. On the way home I determined to pass on further supervised horticultural activity to anyone I could find. And I did, by emphasising the scones and strawberry jam.

The home gardening lark was eventually replaced as my preferred sporting activity by labouring on a building project. Catholic students had been given the chance of paid Wednesday afternoon exercise on the building site for the church's new student hostel, Aquinas Hall. By this time I was a surrogate Catholic anyway through my mates at 2.1.0. They kindly smuggled me onto the construction area with them and we began digging trenches for the standard three bob an hour.

When we arrived, the foundations were in and there were three huts in place. One for the site office, one for the workers and one for tool storage. Piles of timber, bricks and reinforcing steel were scattered about the place in anticipation. Around and among these promises of future activity moved a black, cassock-clad figure topped off with a cloud of grey hair and blessed with a gentle humility. With his legs and feet hidden beneath the priestly robe he seemed to glide effortlessly like a supernatural apparition and looked strangely out of place in this confused landscape of construction. Everywhere he went he was greeted with respectful nods and courteous salutations. Already the church had a presence in place - and that presence was Father McCardle.

He had appeared the same day that the contractors had moved onto to the empty section and had introduced himself as the church's representative, adding reassuringly that he would try to keep out of their way but could he see the quantity surveys? Management had felt obliged to humour him and grudgingly cleared a corner of the tool shed, found a box for a seat and a packing case, turned on its side, as a table. Onto this, with knowing smiles, they had piled the heap of complicated quantity survey calculations. To their surprise they hardly saw him for three days as he religiously ploughed through the papers stacked in front of him.

Eventually he surfaced with the surveys under one arm and a handful of papers covered with calculations in the other and presented himself at the site office with profound apologies for taking so long. He then sat down and, referring to his double-checked figures, pointed out a series of important errors in the quantity estimates for the project.

"That man saved us thousands" explained the foreman as he recounted the episode.

Which explained the new hut on the site furnished with a shiny desk and comfortable chairs for the priest's exclusive use.

Father McCardle was a qualified engineer and an experienced quantity surveyor and had, over the previous twenty years travelled the world, enveloped in a aura of good will, wherever the Catholic Church had a building project. Aquinas Hall was to be his last engagement and his presence was deeply respected and valued by all who were associated with the undertaking.

Today tertiary students face a double whammy. In the eighties casual work, the traditional source of student income, evaporated. In the nineties the mantra of 'user pays' heralded the introduction of student loans tagged with frightening interest rates. The door that the first labour government opened over half a century ago, enabling anyone with the appropriate academic achievement to enter the professions, has now been slammed firmly shut. The cost of living and the cost of study have combined to exclude the children of the poor.

Two of the most expensive university courses today are Medicine and Dentistry - the two professions that the poor most commonly have to turn to. The present generation of young doctors and dentists begin their professional lives facing a double debt - the cost of their education, represented by their student loan, and the cost of entering a practice. All of this can only be recouped through professional fees paid by the public. In effect their *patients* will pay off these debts. Consultation fees will simply rise as the impact of these loans reaches the consulting room and those practitioners not saddled with these commitments will happily fall in line with their indebted colleagues. The user will indeed pay.

It is interesting to look back on the career paths of my contemporaries. Many of those who came from well-to-do families naturally set up their practices in the more affluent communities - they spoke the language of the comfortably off. My working class peers, educated with the assistance of bursaries, tended just as naturally to move into the poorer suburbs or into rural areas - where we also knew the language. This latter group accepted somewhat less income for the perception of a more satisfying and professionally challenging working environment. This is a choice that cannot prove attractive to heavily indebted graduates. Neither rural practice nor service in public hospitals can generate the level of income that will cope with high levels of indebtedness. Thus the present shortage of doctors prepared to work in more remote rural areas, will become compounded.

There is no doubt in my mind that, given today's conditions, I would never have considered medicine as a career and many of my colleagues would have had to make the same decision. I certainly know that Fred Hollows would have been lost to medicine if it meant borrowing money to do so and then having to claw it back from the pockets of the very people he had set out to serve.

Blessed indeed are the meek for they shall inherit what is left.

ON TOUR

Sandwiched between watching postmortems by long distance and trailing around the wards in the wake of the appropriate tutor, we were occasionally treated to bus trips to outlying institutions of care. It was a bit like visiting historic places but less informative.

Built around the turn of the century with castle-like solidity to serve as hospitals for the local community, these buildings had been recycled into long stay establishments when urbanisation drained away the population they originally served. Some were adapted as psychiatric units to house (and occasionally treat) patients suffering from mental illness, while others sheltered patients with physical disabilities that created dependency.

Each of these architectural treasures was set like a jewel in a sea of immaculate lawns bordered by well tended gardens and transcected by sweeping driveways. Scattered about this imposing entrance would be empty seats that few patients would ever occupy. This welcoming prospect offered each new patient and their relatives a false promise of painstaking care and transformation - window dressing that belied the circumstances inside. More could be done with the plants around the institution than could ever be achieved for the patients within in those days.

Sadly this was true of psychiatric care in the fifties. For the restlessly disturbed, sedation was the basic management tool using chloral hydrate and the barbiturates to create a background of zomboid tranquillity. (The tranquilliser drugs, more calming and less sedating, would soon revolutionise this area of psychiatric care.) Intramuscular injections of smelly paraldehyde coped with most acute episodes and failing that the 'straight-jacket' came into its own. This was a canvas, body-length corset wrapped around the thrashing individual, pinning the arms to the sides and secured at the back by a series of attached leather straps pulled through and secured to sewn-on buckles. Patients thus restrained could be released later into a bare cell upholstered on all four walls and the floor, to prevent self harm - the classical padded cell.

It took a Portuguese neurologist, Antonio Monz, inspired no doubt by his nation's penchant for exploration, to introduce the concept of psycho-surgery. His experimental work on chimpanzees gave a surgical colleague, Almedia Lima, the courage to perform the first Pre-frontal Lobotomy in 1935. This surgical approach to the treatment of psychiatric illness enjoyed considerable popularity in the treatment of disturbed, volatile patients (and some cases of severe depression) for several decades, despite the patchy nature of the results. The operation involved cutting those pathways in the brain that linked the Thalamus (a structure deep in the brain between the two hemispheres) with the Frontal Lobes at the front end of each hemisphere.

SHOCKING STUFF

The depressed patient's world is already dulled into profound passivity. Here the catch-cry was 'snap out of it.' An old time remedy was to lower the patient into a pit of snakes - an approach mercifully thwarted in New Zealand by our snake-free policy.

The next popular source of therapeutic shock for psychiatric patients came from Vienna and involved the use of insulin (discovered by Banting, Best and MacLeod in 1921), treating non-diabetic, schizophrenic patients.

Now, diabetics using insulin can enter a state of shock if they take too much of the hormone and too little glucose to balance it. In this situation the falling blood sugar will eventually be insufficient to maintain brain function so that unconsciousness (and even death) may follow. This condition can be rapidly reversed by the administration of glucose.

In 1933 Manfred Sakel claimed success in treating a series of schizophrenic patients by taking them into the unconsciousness of insulin shock and then bringing them out of it by the timely use of glucose. Another tool in psychiatric medicine had been forged and would be used in some quarters for decades to come - again despite uneven results.

U. Cerletti and L. Bini in Rome in 1938 began treating profoundly depressed patients by applying an electric shock across their temples, inducing simultaneous convulsions and unconsciousness. They gave us 'Electro-convulsive Therapy' - E.C.T.

Despite its inescapable associations with mediaeval torture chambers, this procedure did produce enough 'successes' to encourage its continued use. It would have been more acceptable on humanitarian grounds if appropriate anaesthesia had been available. Chloroform had already been abandoned because of its proven liver toxicity and tendency to initiate cardiac arrest, and ether could form explosive mixtures with air that could be ignited by electrical apparatus. Pentothal, the new intravenous barbituate delivered the promise of quick reliable sleep and was then becoming the compassionate touch that had been missing in the E.C.T. room.

However, despite this merciful advance a major complication remained. The violent muscular contractions induced by the shock were sufficient to produce compression fractures of vertebrae in some cases. This remained a steep price to pay for a clinical result that could not be confidently predicted beforehand.

The Indians of South America would soon come to our aid with their poisoned arrows. They gave us Curare and its alkaloids - powerful muscle relaxants that could be reliably reversed. When used in conjunction with Pentothal, Electro-convulsant Therapy would finally have appropriate anaesthesia and a more compassionate face.

Like it or not, E.C.T. sometimes produced very significant and occasionally dramatic improvement in some cases, sparking the hope (for the first time since asylums were established around monasteries in the Fourteenth Century) that the management of severe mental illness could offer more than passive supportive care. This realisation greatly encouraged both the psychiatrists and the nursing staff and introduced a more positive attitude to their daily duties.

Just as E.C.T. was becoming an acceptable tool in the world of psychiatry the much maligned drug companies were developing the first tranquillisers. These would soon overshadow 'shock therapy' and radically change the face of mental health management for the remainder of the twentieth century.

Even as our bus crunched its way along the carefully raked driveway to deposit us on the formal front entrance steps of the asylum the new drugs and improved anaesthetics were still being developed elsewhere. Soon they would be released on this dark mysterious world of mental illness. However, today we would see it as it had been for decades.

The empty foyer was a temple of hope and clean to a fault. Framed, sepia tinted photographs of previous incumbents, their serious faces frozen in another time, looked down from the walls. Tidy potted palms, on the brink of dehydration, struggled to bring the landscape inside and gleaming brass plaques, their messages almost obliterated by compulsive polishing, bore testimony to long forgotten episodes in the history of the building. A place to stand and look, but not touch. Authority was established by heavy varnished doors labelled 'PRIVATE'. A 'welcome' mat would have been obscene. Beyond, dark corridors led to the wards where patients spent their lives and staff their working days.

In a time when Henry Ford said you could have any colour you liked as long as it was black, all hospitals wards and corridors were painted cream and green. When you 'came to' after an accident or an anaesthetic you did not need to ask "where am I" - if the walls were cream and green you knew you were in a hospital. As an article of faith it was never questioned. Furthermore everything made of brass was polished obsessively. Uniformity rules - OK? The walls were cream and green to calm the restless and make the depressed feel at home.

In those days, as far as I could see, psychiatric patients fell into one of three groups. Those who were endlessly restless, those who were enveloped in sluggish depression and those who jumped spontaneously from one extreme to the other - a simple but useful categorisation. In the wards we found all three. It was what went on behind their eyes that interested and eluded me. Crazy but articulate patients always ended up convincing me that they were, in fact, sane - but then salesmen always found me a soft touch as well. I knew I would never make a psychiatrist and this trip would do nothing to change that.

The visit to the E.C.T. room further confirmed that decision. We saw the patient's couch and the varnished mahogany box with the controlling knobs and switches. We anxiously noted the two electrodes, like a pair of slightly flattened ice creams set in black cones anchored to the machine by thick, spirally coiled black wires - and then suddenly we were back in the corridor again. Our guide had hurried us along as though guilty and embarrassed at the same time. We responded by failing to ask a single question. Straight-jackets and padded cells were conveniently omitted from the itinerary and the tour was over.

BACK TO THE FUTURE

Another day, another bus and another tour. This time we visited Kew Hospital, a home for the elderly disabled. For centuries the task of looking after handicapped old folk was placed squarely on the shoulders of the immediate family. Wherever a supportive family existed only the certifiably insane would be granted institutional care. Society, however, would offer shelter and support, on a charitable basis, to those elderly who had outlived their families and were unable to care for themselves. Through an accident of history these dependent individuals were mostly men. From early colonial times New Zealand had attracted single men, especially to the gold fields in the south, the gum fields of the north and farm labourers everywhere else. Many of these remained life long bachelors. Most communities had an 'Old Men's Home' while few had homes for old women. Presumably the women were more self reliant.

A feature of this visit would be the opportunity to learn something of the late stages of what was then called Parkinson's Disease - (Paralysis agitans or The Shaking Palsy) and today is more properly referred to as Parkinson's Syndrome.

James Parkinson (1755 - 1824) first described this condition in a brilliant paper that stood without alteration or addition for over a century. He documented a progressive malady beginning in middle and old age and characterised by stiffening of the body's muscles causing slowness of movement and flexion of all major joints. To this is added a typical, persistent tremor, usually involving the hands. The generalised muscle stiffness made chewing and swallowing difficult and caused accumulated saliva to dribble from the mouth in embarrassing profusion. The patient, bent forward by the stiffened muscles, shuffled along always on the brink of falling forwards. Throughout the long course of this illness the mind usually remained clear - trapped in a stiff and clumsy body.

Kew Hospital cared for a remarkable number of such cases. Many of these Parkinson patients were suffering from a late complication of a viral epidemic (Encephalitis lethargica or Sleeping Sickness) that swept the world about the time of the Great War and has never recurred since.

Treatment had remained virtually unchanged from Dr. Parkinson's day. He had recommended Tincture of Belladonna - extracted from the Belladonna Lilly (known as 'naked ladies' in less polite horticultural circles). This helped dry up the mouth but had little effect on the stiffness. Synthetic compounds based on this ancient recipe were all that could be offered until the early 1970's gave new hope to sufferers.

Within a few years of our visit the survivors of the encephalitis epidemic would have shuffled off to meet their maker. Ironically, within the same time span, patients in psychiatric hospitals would adopt the classical stooped posture and shuffling gate of Parkinson's Syndrome (known as the 'psyco-shuffle') and induced as a side effect of the earlier tranquillisers. In most instances these symptoms would regress on withdrawal of the medication. Recently, however, drug addicts taking 'home bake' morphine have developed a very profound, fulminating and irreversible form of Parkinson's Syndrome caused by a specific impurity that contaminates the product. Jimmy Parkinson would have been impressed.

The other common disability at Kew was the stroke, a condition resulting from the permanent loss of blood supply to a segment of the brain due either to obstruction or rupture of a blood vessel. A bit like a heart attack - only in the brain. They share the same basic causes but have very different outcomes. In both cases the effected tissue dies and is replaced by a scar.

Strokes involving the left side of the brain will effect the right side of the body and vice versa. Thus for naturally right handed people the left side of the brain is dominant and for naturally left hander their right brain is the dominant half. Now the capacity for speech and the ability to read usually lie in the dominant hemisphere. Thus a stroke in the dominant side of the brain may not only incapacitate the dominant arm and hand but may wipe out speech and reading at the same time. The double-wammy is particularly cruel to a mind that knows what is going on and what it wants, but cannot communicate this to the world outside. Adding insult to injury, visitors and sometimes even carers, presume that a person who cannot speak is also either deaf, stupid, or both and address them in a loud voice choosing words that one would select when talking to someone who only had English as a third language.

Strokes involving the dominant hemisphere often increase any tendency towards impatience and aggression and may diminish the inhibitions that are normally imposed on sexual expression. Non-dominant strokes are often associated with a perpetual euphoria linked with a cheerful denial that anything is wrong - an attitude that can make rehabilitation difficult.

The extraordinary thing is that as students we were never taught about these significant emotional handicaps that are faced in some degree by every stroke victim. No attempt was made to get inside the patient's head and look out. Instead we knew the anatomy involved intimately and we presumed we knew it all. Tapping out the patient's tendon reflexes will help with diagnosis but offers nothing towards understanding the struggle that is going on in the mind of the patient. The visit to Kew was an opportunity missed.

A LITTLE TIME OUT

The fifth year of our studies was an oasis in a desert of academic endeavour. This was the year to take a breather and perhaps rediscover a little of the world that lay outside the immediate parameters of the syllabus. With a year free of major examinations most of us took the opportunity to rediscover interests previously neglected through the pressure of work.

Traditionally fifth year students accepted responsibility for the publication of the medical student's magazine, Digest. This annual publication was a sort of who's who spiced with gentle satire and vague social comment all carefully regulated, not by authority, but by the prudence all student commentators must exercise knowing that their eventual graduation still lay in the hands of those whom they chose to chide. Here a pseudonym was no guarantee of anonymity – a lesson I had yet to learn.

In a flurry of overconfidence so characteristic of youth I wrote for Digest a parody of one of the Dean's bacteriology lectures, imitating his labyrinthine delivery and mocking his habit of bearing a stack of reference books onto the podium before each session and then solemnly gathering them up again at the end without ever opening one. Bravely I hid my identity behind the pen name "Koch" – an early pioneer in the role of bacteria as a cause of disease.

The following year, during an oral examination, I found myself facing Sir Charles Hercus – our worthy Dean. In his usual detached way he asked a series of questions with his eyes focussed somewhere in the middle distance. However, just as the session was concluding, he switched his gaze to meet mine in a moment of chilling soul-searching confrontation.

I answered his final question before its significance dawned on me.

"Robert Koch Sir"

"How right you are Parkes – I thought you would know that."

His face resolved into a gentle smile as he wished me all the best for the future. I knew then that I had passed and had been graciously forgiven.

I assisted John Scott to edit the 1954 edition of Digest and Pat Bassett and Fred Hollows supported us. Eventually John would receive a well earned Knighthood and Fred would become a legend in his chosen field of Ophthalmology. Despite the glittering potential of some of the editing team our edition was unspectacular.

Fred and I had a few things in common. We both smoked pipes, shared a cynical view of authority and depended on a government bursary for our medical education. He was a committed communist and the only person I had met who had no intention of gaining personal wealth in this world despite his obvious capacity to do so. His communist philosophy possibly cost him an appointment to a teaching post in Otago Medical School but his acceptance in Australia would eventually lead to his outstanding work with Australian Aboriginal health issues and thence to confront the enormous problems of blindness in the Third World.

He loved mountain climbing and I recall his enthusiastic description of a tall climber he had met somewhere in the Southern Alps. A couple of years later Hilary knocked off Everest and Fred was delighted.

IN THE POO

If fifth year was free of major examinations it did carry one imposition. We were obliged to undertake a public health study and submit a thesis on it. Students were allowed to pair up and John Scott and I made up one such team. All this was a bit of a bind because it took up term holiday time usually devoted to labouring in a brickworks to restore the bank balance.

At the time Auckland was engaged in a battle regarding options for future sewage disposal. One school focussed on the 'Brown's Island Scheme' in which all effluent from greater Auckland would be processed on an island in the Waitamata harbour. The opposing school preferred the Mangere Oxidation Pond scheme.

As it happened I lived in the southwest suburbs, fairly close to Green Bay on the Manukau Harbour and had access to our home built runabout moored there. A few hundred metres down harbour from Green Bay stood an enormous closed-in concrete box, know as 'the septic tank' where all sewage for miles around was held until ebb tide released a tidal gate and the accumulated waste could escape into the harbour. Post war growth of the district meant that this system was now overloaded. Popular myth at the time maintained that during the six hour holding period its contents were magically transformed into an innocuous fluid before release. One's nose seriously questioned this assumption.

Our plan was to gather shellfish adjacent to and downstream from this installation to measure the pollution levels. To do this we needed access to laboratory equipment to culture and incubate the contaminating bacteria. The old Department of Scientific and Industrial Research (DSIR) were very happy to accommodate us as they were already involved in this type of work and access to our results could prove useful to them. While we were arranging this the local Drainage Board got wind of our plans and expressed their interest.

Our rather innocent public health project was beginning to gather political overtones way outside our original proposition. This became more focussed when the Drainage Board learned that we had a boat available from which a study of the outfall could be undertaken. They offered to supply us with a drum of vegetable dye, a series of marker floats and a surveyor to plot the drift.

The plan was to select an early morning high tide and thus catch the first of the outfall and follow it down harbour for six hours until the tide turned again. Fortunately the chosen day was perfectly calm and by about eight a.m. we had the boat positioned in the middle of a black, upwelling mushroom dome of rank sewage about four metres in diameter - resembling a vast cauldron of coffee grounds on a rolling boil. The stench, however, belied this innocent simile.

With half the dye added and surface floats in place we promptly withdrew from the offensive zone and began to plot its down-harbour course while taking water samples at various stages and depths.

Contrary to our expectations the sewage did not disperse laterally at all. The outfall pipe discharged at the very edge of the channel where water flow was much slower than in mid channel. This brisker central flow held the effluent against the shore as we, and it, drifted down with the tide.

Six hours later the ebb was completed and our dyed effluent extended as a sinister band along the inner channel edge for three or four kilometres below the outfall; ending across the entrance to French Bay. With the turn of the tide we all expected the flow to simply reverse and retrace its offensive steps back up harbour but it did no such thing. The rising tide simply moved the sewage inland gently glazing each beach and its shellfish with a layer of human waste.

The realisation that twice each day popular beaches like French Bay and Wood Bay received a generous contribution of effluent from Auckland's south-west suburbs would have shattered property values along this stretch of the harbour. However the full impact of the information age was yet to come and words like 'ecology' and 'environment' had not yet strayed into common usage. Our simple demonstration of the gross inefficiency of such coastal discharge systems would have made compulsive viewing on a T.V. current affairs programme today - but T.V. in New Zealand was a decade away.

The next step was to gather cockles along the path of this outfall and mash them up. A fixed volume of this mollusc puree was then inoculated into a culture medium and incubated at body temperature. The colonies of bacteria that grew were counted and identified (with the help of the DSIR staff). The results, not surprisingly, correlated with the observed passage of the effluent.

At low tide the Manukau Harbour consists of about eighty percent sand banks bordered by deep channels. The sand bank opposite the Green Bay septic tank was a mere fifty metres from the outfall yet the shellfish along that bank were not contaminated -

demonstrating how efficiently the laminar flow in the channel prevented dispersal and held the offending material close to the shore.

Eventually the Drainage Board won the debate and Auckland's human waste was directed to Mangere where oxidation ponds were established to deal with the problem. The scheme imposed considerable discomfort on the local residents before the system operated efficiently. Today the ponds are overloaded and expansion is scheduled.

Future students of Town Planning might like to explore the perverse reasoning that places the effluent of our largest city alongside the airport that welcomes most of our overseas visitors - a bit like putting your toilet by the front door. Wellington managed to maintain their outfall in direct line with their approach runway for decades but have now seen the error of their way. They have finally abandoned this system of disposal and promptly spruced up their terminal building. Now that must be progress.

GO NORTH YOUNG MAN

The temporary easing of academic demand allowed me to read a little medical history, drawing reference books from an obscure corner of the Medical Library. Among a miscellany of books that lacked any specific designation on the shelves I stumbled upon two cheaply bound volumes –"Notes from a Backblocks Hospital" 1938 and "More Notes from a Backblocks Hospital" 1942 – two of the five books written by Dr. GM Smith of Hokianga, Northland New Zealand.

Some years earlier I had seen this giant Scotsman on a picture theatre newsreel when he was denied admission to a meeting in Auckland of the New Zealand Branch of the British Medical Association. His fellow members objected to his dress consisting of open shirt, shorts and sandals. Despite the pleading of his friend Sir Douglas Robb the meeting remained unmoved and Smith, holding doggedly to his sartorial preference, walked away. Here was a man who had worked in remote, poverty stricken Hokianga from 1914 to 1948 – through two world wars separated by a nationwide depression. One of his enduring contributions was the manner in which he organised the medical and nursing services around the hospital, integrating them into a single system. This model, known as a Special Area, was successfully established in several other remote areas of New Zealand and is basically retained today in Hokianga, having survived the allpervading powers of restructuring.

His philosophy of adapting services to prevailing conditions interested me. He argued that the health of any community was intimately associated with an adequate income based on regional development and to this end enthusiastically promoted his own local schemes. The first was to encourage the cultivation of artichokes as a basis for pig farming. The scheme failed when the artichoke crop failed. A later scheme was to turn Hokianga into a tobacco-growing region. Everyone obligingly planted tobacco resulting in an excellent crop. The vast harvest of tobacco leaf was gathered in and hung up to dry wherever appropriate space was available. Within a few weeks the promise of wealth turned to mush as the various moulds and fungi that also thrive in Northland destroyed the crop and the dream.

Through these two books I learned that there were (and still are) 'Outposts of the Empire' within New Zealand where need was a constant state and not a temporary inconvenience. I knew then that I would probably move towards such places but it never occurred to me that I would one day work in his beloved Hokianga.

HENRY'S SADDLE

Sometimes the University Calendar and Easter Weekend conspired to create a longer holiday and on one such occasion I had a chance to join a tramping party and journey between Lake Te Anau and George Sound.

A key member of the party of five was an American student, D.J. who loved our mountains, enjoyed cooking and most important of all owned a sizeable car that would get us from Dunedin to the lake. This was a new experience for me. I had only tramped in the north of the North Island and was usually responsible for organising these ventures. This time I was off the hook. All I had to do was pay my share and follow the others - sheer luxury.

We overnighted in some cabins at Te Anau and gathered on the wharf at dawn next morning for our chartered trip up the lake and along the middle arm. Our vessel was a typical workhorse of a boat - adequate for fifty or so passengers and powerful enough to pull laden barges. I have always loved these solid, no nonsense boats and enthusiastically lead the boarding party.

A draught of warm air, with hot oil on its breath greeted us as we passed the engine hatch. Deep down there a massive diesel engine was being prepared. A series of blow torches focussed on each cylinder head, heating them to ensure an easy and reliable start up. What a delightful way to begin a tramping holiday.

A blast of compressed air eventually urged the pistons into action and with that wonderful deep throated cough peculiar to diesel engines, the motor fired and then settled like a metronome to a perfect beat that comes with good breeding and caring maintenance. Only a slight rise in tempo was necessary to drive us across that glass calm lake. Power without fuss.

The morning was all about mist. Mountains to the west had gathered it modestly about their midrifts, while patchy sheets of fog clung low across the water's surface. As we slid through these it was as though this heavy vessel was gliding through air. Slowly, as though responding to the even throb of our progress, the mist was retreating revealing islands, mountains, headlands and the mirror that faithfully reflected the view.

By slow degrees the skipper, alone in his little glass cage, nudged the wheel to port as we rounded the headland and opened up the middle arm of the lake. The ranges on either side slowly closed in until our wake was caressing either shore, awakening the world to our presence.

Our destination, a small beach at the end of the valley, was now in view. Issues like how we would eventually disembark and reach the shore began to occupy my mind. The launch had neither a dingy aboard nor in tow to act as a ferry and the vessel itself, even when aground, would have water around it up to my armpits. This looked like being a very wet experience - and still we moved closer. Time and again I looked down into the water and each time it remained reassuringly deep - this was not my familiar, shallow, tide-wracked harbour surrounded by low hills and flat land. Here steep cliffs plunged just as steeply into deep water.

With a resting propeller and gently idling motor we glided closer. When only a boat's length from the steeply shelving shore, a short trembling burst of reverse thrust killed our progress just as the bow crunched lightly against the dry pebbles of the beach.

One after the other, like a small family of lemmings, we disappeared over the bow onto the dry shingle beach below, gathered our packs and crunched off without getting our feet wet.

At the edge of the bush D.J. called a halt. As well as his own pack he carried a box of stores - our food for the trip. Each item was carefully labelled. Methodically he divided the largess into five equal piles and then supervised each of us in turn as we stowed our share into our packs. The careful attention he paid to each individual as they found the appropriate space for their share seemed to me to be a case of overdoing things a bit. Later, however, this careful attention would pay off. At meal times he would unerringly approach the correct person for a specific item of food and, if necessary, could also remind them in which part of their pack it had been stowed. I, on the otherhand, had difficulty remembering where I had packed my dry socks.

With the grub supply evenly distributed, we set off up the valley floor and into the bush. The path was remarkably wide and dry. The surrounding trees were mature giants draped in hanging moss and lichen. Grazing deer had kept the undergrowth in check, yielding a park like impression with a floor of moss-covered boulders. Where I had expected a wet, dripping world, I found a strange dryness and commented on it. Steve, the guy who had organised the venture, remarked that the district was currently in the grip of an unprecedented drought and we would need to be especially careful with cooking fires.

Today we attribute the vagaries of our weather to the behaviour of a warm Trans-Pacific current that creates phenomena with cute Spanish names that few can pronounce correctly and less can spell. Fifty years ago we just as firmly believed unpredictable weather was due to atmospheric testing of atomic bombs in the same Pacific Ocean. The atoll that gave us abbreviated swim-wear, Bikini, also gave us contrary weather.

The entire journey would involve three distinct features. The first leg traversed a valley floor including two lakes, the second would be a climb over the ridge via Henry's Saddle and then finally the descent into George Sound. After about an hour's easy tramp along the unusually dry valley floor we reached the first lake.

This narrow, slightly curved lake was beautiful in its simplicity. Bush draped the steep hillsides all the way down to the water's reflecting face. The only hint of human construction to be seen was the inverted dinghy we had arranged to use, tucked away beneath some trees. I wriggled under the boat to look for the tell-tale chinks of daylight that would indicate potentially leaky seams and found none. We had the vessel afloat and loaded, when I made an interesting discovery.

"Who else can row?" I enquired casually.

Four slightly shamefaced companions avoided my gaze - I had my answer.

A quick assessment of the situation suggested that it would take a good hour to row to the head of the lake - unless we could count on wind assistance. Although we stood in the calm of the sheltering trees, there was a distinct wind ripple playing on the lake's surface beyond and that breeze was in our favour. As the sole source of nautical propulsion and slightly drunk with power I took charge and ordered the biggest tent to be unpacked while I secured a suitable sapling for a mast. Using the guy ropes as stays we soon had a functioning rig that caught the friendly wind beautifully and urged us effortlessly up the lake. We slipped along with the gentle grace one could associate with Cleopatra on her burnished throne gliding down the Nile. Bathed in a heady blend of warm sunshine and smug satisfaction I lit my pipe and casually steered with an oar locked in the crook of my knee. Heaven, indeed, is a following wind.

As we neared the head of the lake, like all responsible navigators in uncharted waters, I kept a weather-eye open as we crossed the shallow ground. The lake bottom, a comfortable distance below, was littered with sizeable trout, basking in the flickering sunlight, too comfortable to move as the undulating shadow of our progress crept across them. The primeval bounty of nature innocently awaiting inevitable exploitation.

The voyage completed, we tethered the dinghy to a convenient tree to await our return, and pressed on up the valley. The stream that fed the lake behind us was now much reduced by the recent drought, enabling us to move quite easily up its bed. We made very good time and were soon surprised by an extraordinary sight.

Our second lake had sprung a leak. Like a half empty bath jammed between the hills this smaller lake was even smaller. Bikini, we now realised, had a lot to answer for. The drought had almost dried up the streams that fed it while its waters had percolated away between the rocks that cluttered its outfall. A line of neatly trimmed vegetation, like a kid after a 'pudding basin' haircut, recorded the natural waterline. Below this lay a giant tub lined with dry mud-caked boulders extending down to the present diminished water's edge. The lake was now contracted to about one kilometre in length.

We agreed that although it would be easy to traverse the dry lake bed, it would be prudent to have the boat available for the return trip. One good shower of rain would convert the dry mud that now coated the rocks into a treacherous, slippery surface guaranteed to sprain ankles with casual abandon.

The boat for this leg of the trip was much smaller (after all, someone else had had to drag it here from Lake Te Anau). Unfortunately, instead of being left in the shade, she had been left in the sun, drying out her timbers. All her seams had opened up and some would even need caulking with rag. It would take at least an hour of immersion for the timber to swell and 'take up'. By now matters nautical had become my business and I set about some primitive caulking with rag, scraps of paper and plant fibre pressed into the gaping seams with the back of a sheath-knife.

I was concentrating on this basic task when they attacked - billions of literally blood-thirsty midges and sandflies supported by several squadrons of mosquitos. Our supply of insect repellent (supplied courtesy of some senior chemistry student friends) was seriously challenged - and still they came. I had never experienced an attack like this and resented their imposition while I struggled to complete the task in hand. Suddenly I lost my cool and exploded into an animated and totally ineffective rage.

"Hey guy - don't let 'em get at you psy-cho-logically" D.J.'s quiet voice cautioned from behind.

I turned angrily to rebuke what seemed to be trivialising, banal advice but quickly regained control at the sight of D.J.'s face, swollen beyond recognition and surrounded by his share of insect squadrons. The poor chap was acutely allergic to our attackers and stood there trying to observe me through two slits and addressing me through pale lips engorged with oedema. Suddenly my predicament became very minor by comparison. It began to rain very gently and the attack was over.

By now the timbers of our sunken boat, like poor D.J.'s face, had swollen and the residual leaking was manageable. As soon as she was bailed out I sat amidships with the oars while the others stowed the packs around me. As I rowed up the remnant of the lake, the others scrambled over the rocks before the light rain made their surface slippery and together we arrived at the head of the lake. To complete this stage of the journey all we had to do was drag the boat a hundred or so metres to the trimmed tree edge and secure it.

As we trudged on up the dry stream bed the walls of the valley were closing in. Steve, with his map and compass, was seeking our next focal point - Henry's Saddle. Confidently he struck out towards the western side of the valley and the going became tougher.

It was now more upwards than onwards as we climbed above the tree line and edged our way up the exposed rock face. As climbs go this was a basic straightforward effort. All one needed was a series of alternate hand and foot holds that were conveniently within reach. The trick was to avoid taking a hand hold that the guy above may claim as a foot hold. Squashed fingers were a distinct hazard to happy climbing.

The first attack came when we were within grasping and gasping distance from the top. Like all good fighter pilots they swept in with the sun behind them, turning aside at the very last moment to let fly a torrent of avian abuse and derision. As one kea wheeled away over the valley a second would repeat the pattern forcing everyone to concentrate very carefully on the essential business of hanging on. Perhaps they had a nest nearby - either that or they were just plain bored.

Once we were all safely on the small plateau that Henry had claimed as his saddle, the stroppy keas abandoned their aggressive display and the climbers prepared camp for the night. D.J. as usual, nominated the food required and the names of its bearers together with helpful suggestions on where to find it and a meal was soon underway. We had finished eating when the lone raider attacked. Swooping down in a flurry of feathers, a kea snatched a red plastic cup and was airborne again, sweeping out over the valley in a victory circle as the sun glinted on its prize. Keas 1, Climbers 0.

Oblivion came with the night. I could have dreamed of Cleopatra drifting down the Nile, eating smoked trout - but I was far too tired.

Morning arrived with a rush. It had skipped the poetic preliminaries of dawning to present an instant day that demanded action. Sitting up, I looked out and focussed on a movement in the tussock nearby. Out stalked a weka raising its feet delicately like a house-proud cat walking on wet grass. It spotted a spoon by the fire place, grabbed it in its beak and began dragging it away. The boot I threw at it missed by a mile, but it was enough to inspire a hasty retreat without the booty. Climbers 1, Wekas 0. Lying back I meditated briefly on the kleptomanic tendencies that characterised the bird life that Henry had gathered around him.

Enough! It was time to rise and shine - no matter how dimly. D.J. was already nominating the breakfast ingredients - their carriers and where to find them. Steve, after consulting the map, announced cheerfully that life would be downhill from here - and he was right once again.

Not far from camp we came across a hollow in the rock face, about ten metres across and the same in depth, littered with large broken stones. It was an old mica mine and there were still traces of this special mineral in veins running across the unmined rock face. Whereas we had made an adventure out of travelling this far, the miners (presumably lead by Henry himself) accepted it as part of their livelihood in all weathers.

The easy descent from the saddle to the sound constantly criss-crossed a stream that meandered down the valley. It reminded me of taking a dog or kids for a walk. While you move straight ahead, they rush off to right or left of your path, constantly returning to your line of progress. One moment the stream we were splashing across was running from left to right while at the next crossing it flowed in the opposite direction. It was all a bit confusing but with unshakeable confidence in Steve's compass I followed obediently.

The weeks of rain so recently withheld by the bomb tests were now released in one go as we were nearing the hut on the shore of George Sound. A trickle of water had just breached the protective barrier of my collar and was now snaking its way down my back when the wall of the hut, closely guarded by the trees, came into view.

Thank God for good housekeeping. The previous occupants had left adequate firewood that was now tinder dry. This unwritten tradition that ensures such forethought is a precious aspect of backwoods culture. Happiness is a warm hut with rain drumming on the roof.

And we were happy. Wet clothing steamed away around the fire. There were plenty of bunks and even kerosene lanterns for the evening. By sunset every rain-soaked item was dry while the downpour continued its unbroken hammering outside.

Morning was strangely silent. The rain had stopped and outside you could just hear the muffled gurgling of overfilled streams. My companions had planned a day of rock climbing, but I preferred to stay at sea level. Craggy cliffs may be their element, but salty water was mine.

I had already explored the shore before the climbing party departed. Gathering firewood while the sky was still clear was first priority and quickly fulfilled. The whole shore line was afloat with wood ranging from a myriad of twigs and tangled branches to enormous logs that had rumbled down rivers losing bark and branches on the way. A kind of natural wood processing system that delivered logs, ready for milling, into the waters of the sound.

Among the treasures we found in the hut were a couple of fishing lines. This discovery, coupled with a very rusty tin of lamb's tongues, confirmed my plans for the day. I would go fishing on a Huckleberry Finn raft of logs. By lunchtime the raft was completed and launched onto the calm waters of George Sound.

The fishing was excellent and in due course I had safely landed six good sized blue cod and lost overboard twice that number. Dinner that night was fillet of blue cod pan fried in butter. D.J. awarded me seven out of ten, noting that some segments of lemon and a dash of tartare sauce could have improved the score.

The following day saw us packed and heading back. The return journey was everything one could expect. It seemed shorter, as all journeys do when repeated. The rain stayed away and the ascent to Henry's Saddle was an easier grade. Finally the descent into the valley on the other side would be just that - an easy descent.

We were soon at the old mica mine and then scrambling down from the saddle to the valley below, unchallenged by beak or claw. The only event to mar my personal enjoyment was the sense of something breaking in my pocket as I pressed against the rock face. I had stupidly broken the stem of my favourite pipe.

The recent rain had dramatically transformed the stream that ran in the valley below the saddle. Whereas earlier we had encounted an embarrassed, half starved trickle, we now faced a sizeable stream rushing along impatient with new found energy. We worked our way downstream to confront another transformation.

Our half-empty bath tub of a lake was now brimmingly restored. The dinghy, half-filled with rain water, swung patiently from its tether awaiting our return. We bailed the boat and filled it with packs. While the others worked their way along the tree line I rowed down the lake, dumped the packs and returned to ferry my companions two at a time to the foot of the lake.

At the second lake my luck still held. The wind had conveniently reversed its direction so that with the tent-sail erected we could repeat the Egyptian Princess act. The only thing missing from this victorious performance was a contemplative, celebratory smoke. The remnants of my pipe still lay useless in my pocket.

Once we had stored the boat safely under the trees, D.J., in conference with Steve, conceded that we were well ahead of time and declared a cook-up. We enjoyed a smorgasbord of tinned everything washed down with coffee made the old fashioned way (the age of instant coffee was yet to come).

With slight deference to the sin of gluttony we trudged slowly down the now slippery wet track through the forest of dripping, moss bedraggled trees to emerge beside the lake a good half hour before the launch was due.

Right on time she rounded the headland and surged imperiously towards us. We were ready at the water's edge when her bow nudged the shore to take us on. The whole business had been a model of responsibility, casually arranged and faithfully carried out. The skipper had probably written our arrangements on the back of his tobacco packet, but the system worked. There was no radio with which to tinker with things like E.T.A.'s and cell phones were still part of sci-fi fantasy. They relied on us with the same confidence that we relied on them and now we were heading back to Te Anau as sunset surrendered to evening - as arranged.

As we chugged along the old chap who acted as deck hand and engineer asked me about the trip and as part of my enthusiastic response I mentioned my broken pipe.

"Lets see it," he said and with a 'tut tut' noise he tenderly took my broken offering down to the engine room emerging minutes later with a big smile and my favourite briar restored. Overwhelmed with my good luck and his consummate skill I fumbled for my tobacco pouch and soon had old faithful glowing contentedly. Leaning against the after rail, bathed in the gold of the stern light I puffed the contented puff as the water boiled astern urging us back to Te Anau.

It had been a great trip and perhaps I would dream of Cleopatra and smoked trout or Henry and his thieving birds or George and his blue cod - who knows?

BASIC SHELTER

After functioning for a year as a boarding establishment followed by a similar period as a flat, 2.1.0. broke up and we spread ourselves around Dunedin. Dick, a friend and fellow med. student, had heard of a very basic residence going cheap in the suburbs of St. Clair and together we went out to investigate it.

By this time there was an even greater shortage of student accommodation and all worthy citizens had been urged to help shelter the growing student population. Dunedin, with canny Scots' insight, recognised the value of our contribution to the city's economy and also were justly proud of their founding university. Our eventual landlord, with commendable patriotism, responded to the crisis by offering a humble, two roomed lean-to at the bottom of the section.

This rickety structure had been built as a temporary dwelling many years previously while the house was under construction. When this task had been completed it was retained as a venue for parties until the family, bowed down by domesticity, abandoned regular socialising.

It was a two roomed affair attached to a double brick wall that had been erected along the back boundary of the section. For a few shillings each week we had a shared bedroom and a living - dining - kitchen - study room fortified with yet another practical Shacklock wood and coal burning stove.

Fresh water could be drawn from the garden tap a few metres away and waste water could be flung over the fence into the empty section next door. A toilet, incorporated within the washhouse facilities outside the landlord's house fifty metres away, was accessible at all times and in most weathers. Our agreement to occupy included access to the family home for a bath every Thursday night - even if we did not need one. We happily and gratefully accepted their offer.

Although an outer suburb of Dunedin, St. Clair was an easy level bike ride from the centre of town. Part of this journey passed through the industrial sector and I can still recall the olfactory challenge of the pong of the soap factory followed almost immediately by the sickly sweet smell of chocolate from the home of Cadbury.

My ancient bicycle boasted automatic power transmission. To increase speed one automatically peddled harder. During the modest increase in traffic density that constituted Dunedin's rush hour it was possible to cycle across town faster than the legendary trams could complete the same journey. This advantage came with only slightly increased risk to life and limb. The only significant hazard lay in getting one's front wheel caught in the tram rails. Such an event invariably locked one's direction of progress onto that of any approaching tram, with the consequent increased risk of impact.

Our basic abode had a humble charm based largely on the varied origins of its component parts, a tribute to man's capacity to salvage and recycle. It also exhibited a casual disregard for the fundamental principles of structural engineering. The entire building leaned slightly towards the vacant section behind and the roof sagged gently. It had the comfortable air of a much loved and well worn slipper.

Inside, curtains suspended from the top of the windows fell well outside the window sills as though they had been stiffened to enable them to sustain this jaunty angle. Of course the curtains really hung vertically - it was the wall that leaned. In the world of architecture the Tower of Pisa was not unique.

This list to starboard, it transpired, was not a static phenomenon but was based on the silent dynamics of the brick wall at the back to which the rest of the structure was attached. This wall was very slowly leaning more and more towards the neighbouring property. Technically we lived in a state of dynamic unstable equilibrium.

To calibrate and record this changing condition we set up a plumb bob in the corner of one room and marked, with the dates, its changing position. It seemed to be moving about half an inch per year. Clearly there was some urgency to complete our course of study and move on.

Despite the insidious progression that our shelter was locked into by the force of gravity we were comfortable as long as we could keep the place warm. The problem of heating could be solved by either electricity or coal and wood. Although the former was dear the latter was cheap. Furthermore, he who chops his own wood is twice warmed. Firing up the stove provided a system of central heating that was adequate although thermodynamically inefficient. With the oven door open we had access to a wonderful foot warmer.

At first the traditional weekend roast posed a problem. Sometimes it would be cooked within a couple of hours and at other times Mr. Shacklock's product would take three times as long to perform the same task. This perverse property made predicting meal times a very difficult business until we eventually tumbled on the solution by combining climatic data with combustion technology. A good southerly wind (about 4 to 6 on the Beaufort Scale) would so improve the draught through the stove that a leg of mutton would be cremated very quickly if not watched carefully. Winds of whatever strength from the north contributed nothing to the thermal efficiency and the offering would cook long and slow. Thus by including weather information in our database it became possible to schedule meal times with satisfactory precision.

These were the days when the domestic electricity supply was used for all lighting, some cooking and occasional heating. The available range of electrical appliances was still limited and wall outlets (still two-pin plug affairs) were uncommon. This lack of wall sockets led to the imaginative and dangerous use of light fixtures as the main access to power. The popularity of 'meccano' sets as toys for boys lead to a male population subconsciously conditioned to assemble complex structures from basic units. Thus one light fitting could become the source of power for any number of appliances provided the relevant fuses had been suitably reinforced to carry the load. The robust nature of house wiring in those days probably explained the relative rarity of house fires attributed to electrical overload.

The friendly corner shop supplied the ingredients for most meals at a time when refrigeration was a rare domestic phenomenon. Our corner store was run by a pleasant chap with a good supply of fresh vegetables and more than a passing interest in our nutritional intake. Once when purchasing peas in the pod to enhance the weekend roast he treated me to his wild vision of the future. He confidently predicted that peas in the pod would soon be a thing of the past to be replaced by packets of frozen shelled peas that one would take home to store in a unit called a deep freeze. I was sure that his imagination had finally run amok.

The last two years of study in Dunedin passed pleasantly and affordably, thanks to the modest rent involved. We could even treat friends to the occasional meal provided the strength and direction of the wind could be reliably forecast.

Despite the slow subsidence of our dwelling (which worried the landlord when he saw the irrefutable evidence of our plumb bob) we enjoyed our time and remain grateful to the generous spirit that inspired the Dunedin public to support and tolerate the transient student population, despite the occasional lapses in behaviour and taste that characterised our life style.

FEVER

During the summer vacation that separates fifth year from sixth year, medical students were scattered around the country for what today is called 'work experience'. That was the theory. In practice the nation was so short of junior doctors that most of us ended up as unofficial house surgeons, replacing the regular appointees during their holidays - it was heady stuff. In recognition of our novel though temporary status we wore the coveted long white coats, received a modest (though welcome) allowance and desperately tried not to blush when addressed as 'doctor'.

I found myself draughted into the Infectious Diseases Block at Auckland Hospital. This establishment had evolved from the Fever Hospitals of the previous century. In that bygone era hospitals - particularly Fever Hospitals - were always sited on hills to escape what was believed to be the unhealthy atmosphere of the valleys. In New Zealand our pioneer forebears carefully placed most of our hospitals overlooking the towns they served. It is as well they did. Today smog and pollution fulfil the role that earlier generations wrongly attributed to the gentle morning mist.

The role of the Fever Hospital was to isolate infectious patients from the population in general and from inpatients with more worthy ailments. Infectious diseases were usually accompanied by high temperatures, were often untreatable and frequently fatal. Any fever without an identified cause had to be treated as though it was an infectious disease until proven otherwise.

The Auckland Infectious Disease Unit was a fairly modern three storied affair pushed away to the edge of the hospital grounds and built down a steep bank so that the top floor was at road level. The entire establishment was known as Ward 22, A, B and C.

With my newly issued long white coat draped casually over my arm I set out to explore the new world on my horizon and I was greatly relieved to find the regular House Surgeon was still on duty and deeply concerned to learn that he would be leaving in a couple of days. He showed me where to hang up my long white coat - permanently - here we would wear special gowns like everyone else in the unit. There would be none of the popular movie image of doctors surging down corridors with unbuttoned coats billowing out in a display of dynamic authority reminiscent of the courting rituals of peacocks.

This was the Infectious Block where diseases could be caught and spread. We were not the hospital's untouchables - but folk in the know tended to stand back just a little.

The top floor, Ward 22A, had an admission room in the middle and specialised units at either extremity of the ward. The first of these contained the 'iron lung'. Here a patient with respiratory paralysis from poliomyelitis lay partially engulfed in a long rectangular metal box. Her head protruded through a diaphram that sealed around her neck while her feet emerged from the other end. The whole thing looked like a tiny flat-sided submarine with a series of port holes along each side, so arranged that nurses could attend to the patient's basic needs. A confusion of pipes and cables, punctuated with various gauges, entered and emerged from the apparatus and then centred around a small electric pump which rhythmically raised and lowered the air pressure inside, thus substituting for her failed respiratory capacity - the thing made her body breath.

Overwhelmed by the shear complexity of the machine I hastily confessed my total ignorance of Lord Nuffield's gift to every hospital in the Empire.

"Don't worry old chap, the nurses know all about it - and anyway she can almost manage without it and could be out of it soon".

To my immense relief, two days later she had been successfully weaned from the contraption.

At the opposite end of 22A was a three roomed suite dedicated to diphtheria patients. The first room was a tiny adult bedroom.

"You'll have to sleep here whenever you have a case liable to go into respiratory obstruction".

The middle room was the patient's nursing unit.

Finally he showed me through the miniature operating theatre where the life saving tracheostomy would be performed by the first on the scene able to do so. He showed me where the sterile instruments were stored and gave me a crash course on the procedure.

"You'll need two nurses. One at the top holding the head extended back over the end of the table with the chin in the midline. The second nurse holds the kid's arms down with her elbows across the chest. Now locate the trachea between thumb and finger with the left hand and stick your knife in half way between the sternal notch and larynx - for Christ sake don't cut into the larynx. Now stuff a pair of Spencer-Wells in and open the wound. The kid will suddenly breath with a hiss and a roar, spraying diphtheria over you and everyone else. Now stuff in the tracheostomy tube and tie it in place with a tape around the neck. Got it - good 'cos its tea time."

After tea it was lumber puncture time.

All cases of meningitis, both proven and suspected, were admitted to the unit and lumber punctures were a way of life for us all. The antibiotic streptomycin had just begun to change tuberculous meningitis from being invariably fatal to a condition associated with a reasonable chance of some sort of survival. Patients benefiting from this improved prognosis paid for it through repeated lumbar punctures as this was the only way the management of the disease could be adjusted. Mercifully the intense headaches that characterised the condition were usually relieved for the meantime by lumbar puncture through the consequent lowering of pressure within the skull.

Fortunately for me and the patients my mentor was a good teacher. He knew how to marshal the important practical issues and deliver the information in a way that I could absorb. That morning we had six cases of T.B. Meningitis due for a lumbar puncture and by lunch time I had the hang of it, thanks to a competent tutor, and some trusting patients.

Ward 22C - the one at ground level at the bottom of the hill - was dedicated to all cases that involved diarrhoea. The nursing staff there were brilliant at getting fluid into babies and others with only occasional recourse to intravenous drips.

Before each wardround the nursing staff would have secured the latest soiled nappy from each babe and lined them up, all suitably labelled, for the doctors to examine. Some doctors maintained that they could manage cases purely on the evidence presented in this way. I, however, never discovered the secret. The whole smelly business brought to mind a light hearted article in a medical journal of that time entitled "The Lost Art of Stool Gazing". The author and I shared the same scepticism.

One would hardly expect a ward full of patients with diarrhoea to attract much in the way of drama yet 22C managed to do so twice during the time I worked there.

The first occasion involved pure chaos. A dozen or so prisoners at nearby Mt. Eden Prison had managed to get hold of a pumpkin and cut a hole in the top through which they had evacuated all the seeds and replaced them with sugar. The violated vegetable was then concealed under a pile of shavings in the woodwork room in the hope that it would eventually yield pumpkin wine - which it did. However the brew was contaminated, probably with a tasteless staphylococcal toxin.

The pumpkin's tainted bounty was generously shared among everyone on the wing but after a latent period of about two hours the revellers were all attacked by simultaneous vomiting and diarrhoea. A stream of ambulances and paddy wagons sped them all to 22C with all the drama of a major breakout.

The building was infested with guards and police reinforcements while the wretched prisoners lay helpless on the floor. An army of nurses valiantly tended to the fundamental problem.

Like a tropical downpour it was all over as suddenly as it had begun and within twenty four hours the ward was back to normal and a dozen weak exhausted individuals were safely back behind bars.

At any one time the ward would have at least one case of typhoid fever. Now the word typhoid is derived from the Greek word 'typhos' which means cloudy or smokey and refers to the state of mind frequently encountered in the disease.

We had a middle-aged Maori chap with typhoid and the fluctuating high temperature that usually goes with it. He had been isolated in a single room and his mind was certainly cloudy. Late one afternoon he simply disappeared. It was dark, cold and raining by the time a reluctant police search was launched.

Once again the building was crawling with constables but there was an obvious reluctance to begin searching the bush that surrounded the unit. They probably would have been happier if their quarry had been an armed offender instead of a case of typhoid fever. Our reassurances regarding their future health, should they touch him were clearly inadequate. Eventually we struck a deal. If they found him we would bring him back to the ward. With this treaty in place the search began.

After a couple of hours searching through damp bush with torches two of the searchers literally stumbled on him buried under a heap of leaves that he had piled over himself in a vain attempt to stay dry and warm. The poor fellow clung to his rescuers with such desperate tenacity that they had no option but escort him back to safety.

While their relieved colleagues went off to get them a change of clothes our reluctant heroes were treated to a hot bath with the most pungent antiseptic soap we could find - a gesture that had more to do with public relations than infectious disease risk management.

The patient, now safely back in his isolation room (with the window securely locked) made such a good recovery that one pondered the possible therapeutic value of rotting leaves.

The visiting consultant to the unit was Dr. Hughes, known affectionately to all as 'Katie' (but never to her face). She was a woman of generous proportions who none the less got around in a Morris Minor car. Katie was one of those brave and determined women who had pioneered a place for her sex within the profession and sustained her right to be there with natural dignity.

We had a young lady in the unit suffering from leprosy. She was a Pacific Islander with a limited command of English and was due to be transferred back home to a leprosarium. Katie had taken her shopping for appropriate clothes before the voyage - and probably paid for them herself. Sometime later a thank you letter arrived at the unit addressed to 'Dr. Huge c/o Ward 22'. It stood in the letter rack for some time before Katie claimed it with a smile.

All cases of meningitis in the Auckland District were treated in the unit. Tuberculous meningitis was still depressingly common but the most common of all was meningococcal meningitis. Given massive doses of penicillin supported by one of the soluble sulpha drugs many of these cases would survive. The teaching at the time was that overcrowded housing was the primary factor that accounted for the prevalence of most infectious diseases - particularly T.B., gastroenteritis and meningitis. In the paediatric unit our fellow physicians equated the alarming incidence of acute rheumatic fever with poor housing. Medical Officers of Health also agreed. Fifty years later nothing has changed - some still have third world housing and the diseases that go with it.

From time to time overseas nurses visiting New Zealand on working holidays would find temporary employment in the unit. An American nurse, with a droll turn of phrase, made quite an impression. Her first job was to bath a polio patient and was told to use the thermometer in the bathroom to check the water temperature.

The instrument in question was a floating dairy thermometer designed to measure the temperature of milk throughout a variety of processes. It was so ballasted that it would float upright. However our version had been around for a while and most of its calibrations had worn away.

"You know", she said, "You colonials sure are weird - I had to bath that polio but I couldn't read your God damn thermometer - at one place it said 'butter' and another place 'cheese' - so I bathed him half way between butter and cheese and he did just fine."

I arrived on 22B one morning after a day off to find the entire staff wearing fluffy slippers while here and there were notices requesting 'Quiet Please'. Every door had a short thick fabric belt extending from one door handle, across the edge of the door and secured to the other handle, effectively stopping the door from fully closing.

The ward sister volunteered the answer. In a quiet voice she explained - "We've got a query tetanus."

During the previous evening the night staff had admitted a lad of about eight years. He lay in a darkened room while the entire ward tip-toed quietly about their duties. Even the busy clang and clatter of the sluice room was stilled.

Thanks to almost universal immunisation against tetanus this disease was already rare amongst children. The tetanus bug produces an incredibly powerful toxin, even from an apparently trivial infection. This toxin causes the muscles of the body to tighten up and the resultant stiffness shows up most obviously in the contracted jaw muscles (hence 'Lock jaw'). Sudden noise can so stimulate the patient that all muscles contract further, causing the body to arch backwards in a painful spasm. Each episode would contribute further to the patient's exhaustion.

Good nursing supported by medication and adequate sedation saw the lad home again within a month.

The strangest experience of my tour of duty came near its end.

Late one afternoon I was called to admit a case of malaria. He was a Pacific Islander in his mid twenties who had contracted malaria in Indonesia. This episode was simply a relapse characteristic of the illness. He could have been managed at home but he lived in a boarding house and his landlady was both adamant and terrified.

To confirm the diagnosis the policy was to monitor the temperature and take a blood sample as the fever peaked. After that the appropriate medication could begin while we awaited laboratory confirmation. These arrangements were in place when the Ward Sister informed me that we always notified Carrington Psychiatric Hospital when we had a case of malaria. Doubtfully I rang them and they were delighted. Could I please hold back on medication and they would be around shortly.

I had just taken the blood sample from a now violently shaking, sweat soaked patient when a doctor with two attendants escorted a middle aged man who shuffled along with a peculiar stamping walk. Sister directed them to a side room.

Their plan was to inject some of my patient's malaria packed blood into the backside of their patient in the hope that he would contract malaria. With laboratory confirmation of the diagnosis they loaded a syringe from the sample and advanced down the corridor.

Their man was suffering the late stages of syphilis and was in the grip of classical 'delusions of grandeur'. He sat there, dressed in an odd assortment of ill fitting clothes. Staring into the middle distance he addressed an imaginary bevy of hand maidens. His gently modulated voice thanked one for his slippers and called on another for a cup of tea.

"Two sugars m'dear - thank you - now Mary is dinner ready?"

And so it flowed, unbroken even by the injection. How grand indeed were his delusions and how comforting.

Syphilis had virtually been eradicated by penicillin some years before but the causative organism, once it was established in the brain seemed to be somehow sheltered from the antibiotic. It was however, acutely sensitive to extreme elevation of body temperature and the fever induced by the malaria was often sufficient to push the illness into remission. After a few feverish rigors his malaria would be treated.

I saw him a few weeks later when his delusions had lost their grandeur. You could certainly call it a remission. He sat slumped in a chair silently looking out of the window - perhaps dreaming of his lost harem and the comfort they had so tirelessly dispensed.

AN END AND A BEGINNING

For our sixth and final year of study we were assigned to those major hospitals that were linked to the Otago Medical School by an established clinical teaching unit. After a few weeks of long - white - coated glory we were students again, bringing up the rear of endless wardrounds.

This archaic ritual dates back to the first hospitals of the late sixteenth century when some physicians generously gave part of their time to charitable causes without fee. In recognition of their sacrifice they were treated with the degree of pomp and ceremony deemed appropriate to the level of their philanthropy.

By now paid appointments had replaced the honorary system and the present incumbents were known as 'Consultants' though they still expected (and received) the pedantic adulation of yesteryear.

The hierarchy of the wardround was clearly defined and well understood. The Consultant and Junior Specialist took the lead while Ward Sister rode 'shot-gun', anxiously darting about checking that nothing could obtrude on the dignity of the occasion. Behind them, maintaining a discrete distance, came the Registrar and Housesurgeon clutching notebooks and clinical records. They were followed by the Physiotherapist and Occupational Therapist and we students formed a gaggle at the rear, invariably out of step. The only thing missing was a brass band playing a stirring tune.

For the patient the visitation crowded around the bedside was a milestone in the history of their illness. A word from the besuited oracle could enable them to arise from their bed and walk - or condemn them to a longer stay.

Many Consultants sneered at any hospital smaller than Auckland's. If General Practice, in their view, occupied the bottom of the professional barrel then a career in a country hospital was little better.

"Here's another case that languished in a country hospital", was a common bedside introduction to a new case. I found this attitude to lesser worlds distasteful - particularly as I suspected that I could end up in either. As it turned out I did both.

The shortage of junior medical staff was such that from time to time those of us who had already worked as substitute housesurgeons were occasionally invited to go back and work in our old stamping grounds. These interludes brightened up what was otherwise a tedious and relatively unproductive year.

In some specialities there was also a shortage of Consultants that dated back to the war years. Opthalmologists were in short supply in Auckland and previous incumbents were invited to come out of retirement and serve in the Eye Department clinics. One such elderly gentleman helped out for a couple of afternoons a week. However he had a frustrating habit of mysteriously disappearing for an hour or so, reappearing later to continue the consultations.

The nursing staff were both frustrated and baffled by this pattern of events. On one such occasion it was decided to reassess the waiting patients in the hope that some of them could be referred to a more junior doctor and thus relieve the congestion.

The nurse engaged in this exercise moved among the waiting patients checking names against records until she reached an old chap asleep in the corner with his hat pulled down concealing his face. She gently raised the hat and apologised profusely having solved the mystery.

Many of our clinical teachers were excellent but all presumed that we would be following in their speciality and would soon be booking a trip to the U.K. for post graduate studies. They constantly overlooked the fact that only twenty percent of any class would eventually do that. Eighty percent would enter some form of General Practice, yet in six years of study we had spent about six hours with a G.P. We knew a lot about rare conditions that we might never see again but had little idea what measles looked like or how to identify and treat scabies.

This glaring omission would eventually be corrected when a second medical school was established in Auckland and both schools belatedly recognised the value of a syllabus that recognised Family Medicine as the speciality that it really was. Full credit must be given to those who pioneered that transformation.

Suddenly it was all over. The course had been completed and the class, like migrating birds, was drawn back to Dunedin for a brisk few weeks of final examinations, a quick Graduation Ceremony (which included a passing nod to Hippocrates) followed by sudden spontaneous dispersal.

We now held 'Provisional Registration', enabling us to work under supervision in hospitals for a year before we could apply for 'Full Registration' as medical practitioners. Between graduation and serving once more as housesurgeons most of the class plunged into matrimony. The title 'doctor' was now borne without the slightest blush. We had made it.

My first few weeks as a genuine Housesurgeon were spent in Casualty. The word dates back to Middle English and served well at the time. Later, when 'patients' became 'clients' and the casual breaking of bones and perforating of skin escalated to include the crushing of entire bodies by new and enormous forces, rebranding was demanded and 'Accident and Emergency' was born.

The first morning - a Monday - promised a quiet beginning. The trauma of the weekend had already been tidied up and the city had not been back at work long enough to damage itself. The first couple of hours passed quietly with minor tasks. I had just finished a bit of suturing when a senior nurse popped her head through the cubicle's curtains and in an urgent whisper directed me to attend room seven as soon as possible.

This was it. With drying mouth and quickening pulse I hurried off in search of room seven and the unknown trauma it contained - could I cope? Truth was I only knew of six rooms and was passing the tea room in search of the seventh when a voice called out in that resigned tone reserved for the ultimate in stupidity - "In here - tea or coffee."

The initiation was now completed and a cup of coffee ushered me into the circle of real doctors and nurses. It was the 'fair beginning of a time' and later I applied for a job at Whangarei Hospital.

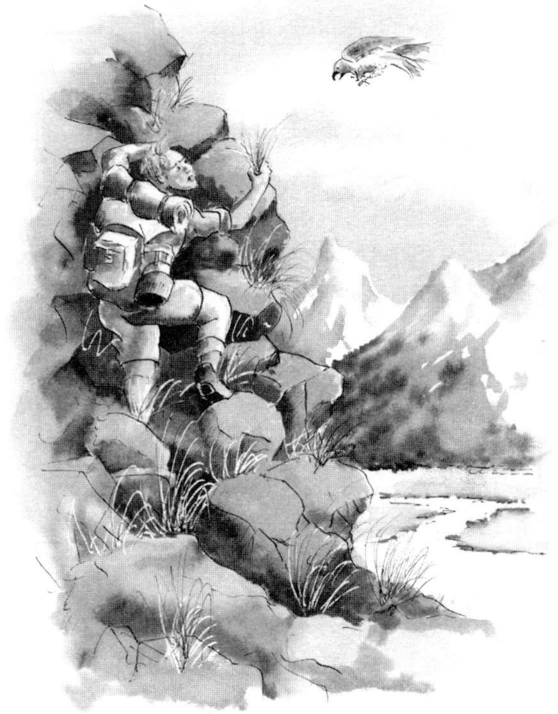

Adventures on Henry's saddle.

NEVER TIE YOUR SHOES WITH FLAX

If you tie your shoes with flax you are doomed never to leave the North
- A common saying on the gumfields of the North.

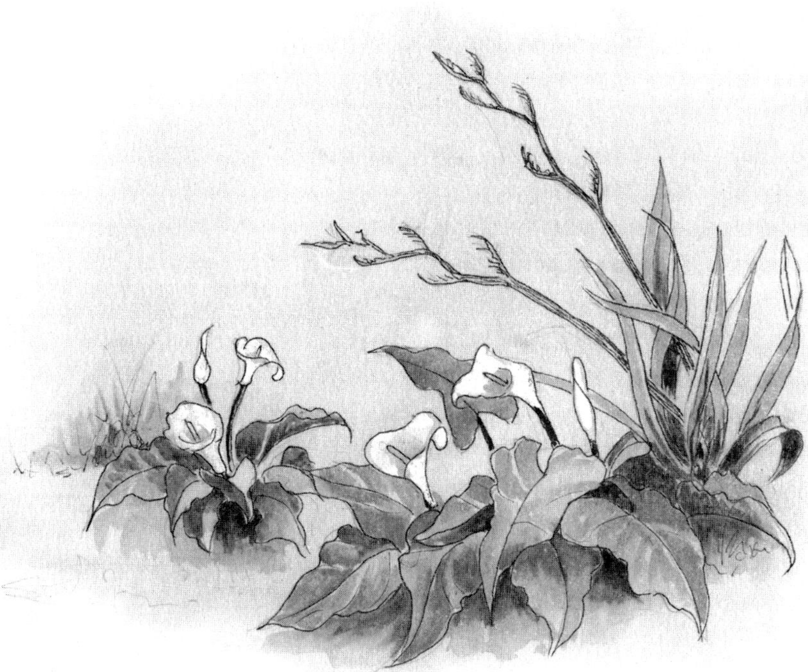

WHANGAREI

In the late fifties the Borough of Whangarei was a scraggy, pimply, adolescent town, simultaneously arrogant in its isolation, yet unsure of its real place in the scheme of things. It could have passed as an unexceptional borough of Auckland had it not been separated from that paternal metropolis by nearly five hours of dusty driving over narrow, unsealed tortured roads. It was this isolation that bestowed its particular claim to fame. In the Province of North Auckland, Whangarei was the biggest fish in a big, though very shallow, pond.

The town, originally nourished by a maritime link with Auckland, had grown up like a ring of mushrooms around its port. Later the railway would successfully challenge the sea as the all-providing umbilical cord and draw future development up various river valleys that still continue to flood one at a time or all at once and at regular intervals.

By depositing coal, limestone and fire-clay about its periphery, nature had been kind to Whangarei. At first the lime was used solely to support grass growth in the pioneering days of farming, while the coal provided domestic and exportable energy. Later these two were combined in the manufacture of Portland Cement and further coal was consumed to fuel a productive brick-works. The supply of coal faded out in the late fifties when the last functioning mine flooded, leaving the cement works to rely on coal shipped into the district from the South Island.

This rhythm of boom and bust would continue to haunt the district throughout the second half of the century as various enterprises flourished and collapsed. Throughout this history of fluctuating prosperity, three industries remained reasonably stable - farming, boat building and cement production. The Marsden Point Oil Refinery proved to be a mixed blessing. Its construction generated a short lived burst of local prosperity followed later, during its expansion, by an even greater flurry of employment punctuated by some of the worst industrial strife that this nation had seen. The refinery today offers a reliable background of wage cheques to a small steady work force.

When I arrived in 1956 no one had dreamed of an oil refinery in New Zealand, let alone in Whangarei. The town was a borough impatient with city aspirations. However it did have a hospital, which by then had become the flagship to the small flotilla of country hospitals dotted about the north. Furthermore its immediate future was automatically assured by its distance from Auckland. Anyone sick enough to require transport to a bigger centre was too sick to make the long, exhausting road journey. Air ambulances were becoming a reality in back-blocks Australia, but no where else.

I found the hospital where all good hospitals should be - at the edge of the town, elevated above the morning mists and spread out to catch the healing rays of the sun. It was a single storied structure of local kauri with a long wide corridor at the back, from which the various wards sprang forward like so many glass-sided fingers extending out clasping the hillside. A small T.B. shelter stood discreetly alone to the right, while a maternity unit, appropriately detached from the main hospital, overlooked it from behind while occupying a world of its own. The nurses' home, a multi-storied ferro-concrete affair of recent construction, was linked to the main hospital by a covered walkway. This, the most modern building on the site, harked back to medieval times in concept. It consisted of a warren of tiny monastic cells each allocated as private living space to a female member of the nursing staff. A solo sailor in a tiny boat enjoyed more personal space.

From the road below, a long concrete path, wide enough to accommodate a brass band in marching formation, ascended the hillside straight to the hospital's centrally located front door. The grade was such that its progress was interrupted at intervals by short flights of steps that accelerated ascension to the next level. The whole thing reminded me of a series of locks on a European canal - which was rather surprising because I had never been to Europe. Prudent locals drove their cars around to the back of the institution to gain easier access, leaving the more formal frontal approach to the young and fit or to first-time out-of-town visitors. Van Gogh would have loved the pair of cypress trees that stood as silent sentries half way up.

Determined to make a grand entry, I strode up the path with a contrived air of confidence, which I hoped concealed the nervous anticipation that always accompanies the first day at a new job and soon found myself face to face with the boss, Clive Lambert, a short nuggety, quietly spoken man in his mid fifties, who looked and moved like a prize fighter. His sole expression of surprise or incredulity was 'crikey', which had earned him his nick-name. The respect of his peers came from his technical competence and his instinct to rely on common sense and experience above science as the basis for his surgical judgement. He was an unpretentious surgeon of the old school who had gathered around him a small team of younger specialists, who were already expanding the scope of the hospital.

With three short sentences he welcomed me, advised me to be on duty the next day at eight a.m. and warned me that my duties could include service at any of the Board's peripheral hospitals. He then handed me over to the House Manager, Mr. Leadbeater, to sort out such mundane matters as accommodation and salary.

Mr. Leadbeater reminded me of a one-man-band, consistently playing several instruments at once. Somehow he kept track of all hospital supplies, staff pay and even repairs to broken toasters. Each fortnight he would wander the corridors of the institution armed with a large, shallow, cardboard box packed with small, labelled brown paper envelopes containing the appropriate coin of the realm - wage packets. One would be stopped in full flight anywhere in the building and offered with one hand the earnings accumulated over the past two weeks together with a demand for immediate settlement of any outstanding debts. A colleague memorably summed up the situation with the observation -

"Here comes Mr. Leadbeater, dishing out the pay as though it was made from his own haemoglobin!"

Our House Manager had his critics, but it eventually took quite a team to replace him and a lot longer to get a toaster repaired.

The Hospital Board, with commendable foresight, had recently erected two double-flats to accommodate the junior medical staff (three House Surgeons and a Junior Registrar). This innovation successfully ensured that the hospital attracted sufficient applications each year - but it did not quite compensate for the requirement to work two weekends in every three and in those days weekends began at noon on Saturday. However, time off in small hospitals was more notional than real and this applied as much to the senior staff as to their junior colleagues.

I began my duties in Whangarei on the surgical run working under Crikey and Bob Mulligan, the second General Surgeon. From the point of view of age they could have been father and son - but the analogy stopped there. Crikey, ever conscious of the burden of responsibility that he carried as Superintendent, found himself trapped in a stifling aura of authority that he found difficult to shake off. He had the boxer's instinct to keep up his guard at all times. Bob, on the other hand, enjoyed every moment of every day and shared this enthusiasm for life with everyone around him. For the humble Junior House Surgeon they made a great team.

Manual dexterity in a surgeon must be matched with sound judgement. One without the other can spell disaster. Crikey, backed by years of experience as a solo surgeon in small hospitals, had both and rarely relied on laboratory tests to confirm his decisions. As a tenderfoot in a field of booby traps I found his instinct for the correct course of action fascinating. When Clive Lambert was on call, all he wanted to know was that a new patient had arrived. He didn't appreciate a dissertation on the relevant laboratory tests, he simply wanted to see the patient for himself. A few questions, a prod of the tummy and a look at the tongue and he would wander off to attend to a dripping tap, a squeaky door or a broken window catch.

"Crikey," he would say. "It smells like an appendix to me."

"But the white count is normal, and ..."

"Shall we say theatre in an hour - and I'll get a screwdriver to fix that window."

With a flurry of quick, precise movements the offending organ would soon lie in a kidney dish and preparations would begin to close the belly. As his assistant you were usually more nuisance than help, but he always acknowledged your presence by offering something safe for you to hold while he got on with the operation. At 'close-up' time inattentive house surgeons had been known to find the fingers of their gloves sewn into the wound.

BLOOD

If house surgeons had little time off, sole charge laboratory technicians had even less. Whenever they left home on evenings and weekends they were obliged to leave a string of contact telephone numbers that would account for their every move. A truly private life for them was out of the question.

In addition to performing a raft of tests, they were also responsible for the blood donor service. Before the days of blood banks this precious fluid was kept warm and on-the-hoof until called for. Each laboratory had a list of prospective donors and their blood types, together with their contact phone numbers. Having surrendered a pint of the best, the unselfish citizen was routinely offered the choice of a cup of tea and a biscuit or a generous shot of brandy before driving home - nobody wanted them to faint while at the wheel - such was our concern for road safety.

My attention had been drawn to the value of early blood transfusion in burns cases. This new imperative was based on the observation that during the burning process millions of red blood cells were irreparably damaged as they surged through the area of intense heat, later precipitating a detrimental level of anaemia.

Consequently, when a badly burnt child was admitted one Saturday night I called for a pint of blood. Now Saturday nights were always bad-news nights for blood donor services. This was the night of maximum trauma coupled with the very time that many donors would be out on the town and difficult to trace.

Impressed by the novel logic of the new burns policy, our Lab Technician responded enthusiastically to my request and began an intensive ring-around as soon as the child's blood type had been determined. Some time later he triumphantly entered the ward clutching a small warm bottle of blood and emphasised the great trouble he had experienced in tracking down a suitable donor. I grasped his offering gratefully and we soon had a red stream dripping into a very distressed and restless child.

The response, within a few minutes, was dramatic. The child quickly settled down and to the amazement of the nursing staff, slept peacefully for the next eight hours. Clearly we had witnessed a modern miracle in burns management. Next morning I called into the Lab to share the extraordinary success of the early transfusion policy with the technician.

"I'm not surprised - I only had one compatible donor on my list and I eventually found him at a party - he was pissed out of his mind - has the kid got a hangover?"

I recalled this incident many years later when alcohol drips were briefly promoted as a sure-fire way to stop premature labour in the Maternity Ward.

Bob Mulligan was on call the night I admitted a very sick bloke haemorrhaging from a peptic ulcer. These are tricky cases because they have always lost a lot of blood before they reach hospital. As they sink into shock, their blood pressure falls and the bleeding eases, but at this stage they are now unfit for surgery. Following a transfusion the pressure will rise again, often triggering further haemorrhage. It takes a bit of juggling to catch them on the rise and move them into theatre before they sink back into a parlous state once more. It is always unwise to operate without some extra blood on hand and it was my job to chase that extra pint.

Earlier in the evening the lab chap had bled a compatible O negative donor - the only one currently available on his list. The patient belonged to a fairly rare blood group and the hunt was now on to find a suitable second donor. As the first pint trickled in and the night wore on I made regular visits to the lab to encourage progress. Meanwhile the patient lingered precariously in a state that was only just appropriate for surgery.

"I've found a suitable donor - come back in about twenty minutes."

This is what we all wanted to hear and with everyone poised for action I returned through the darkened corridors to the laboratory at the appointed time. The only light in the place shone over the couch where donors lay during the procedure. On the plinth relaxed the technician, casually reading a magazine held in one hand, while his other arm was extended along the mattress. A length of tubing connected it to a bottle on the floor, which was already nearly full of blood.

It was a crazy thing to do. Had he fainted during the procedure he would have simply gone on bleeding. The old fashioned blood bottles had a vent to release the air displaced as the bottle filled. Once the bottle was full, blood would have escaped through the vent and onto the floor. On the other hand we could now proceed - and the patient never looked back. That technician had certainly earned his brandy.

SOLVING A MYSTERY

I had wandered into the X Ray Department in search of Crikey and found him immersed in an animated discussion with a bevy of long white coats, representing every speciality in the place. At the centre of their attention was a strange chest x-ray, silently a-glow on the viewing screen like an exotic art treasure in a darkened gallery.

The issue under debate was the grossly elevated right diaphragm. Was it pushed up by a mass in or just above the liver or was the lesion inside the chest space and actually above the diaphragm? Opinion was equally divided and strongly expressed. Irrespective of the position of the diaphragm, what the hell could the mass be? A string of possible pathologies had been enunciated covering most of the contents of Boyd's Textbook of Pathology - but in the end nobody had it right.

Suddenly, ignoring the disputation bouncing around him, Crikey walked up to the film and solemnly counted the ribs down from the top selecting one which overlay the centre of the mass.

"Remember that Parkes - ninth rib. We'll have a look under local after lunch."

"Crikey" I thought and went off to make the necessary arrangements.

The patient harbouring the mystery was a rather shrivelled up old chap with a quick wit and a slow body. He could become breathless just listening to the races on the radio. The choice of local anaesthetic was really no choice at all - this man was certainly unfit for the type of general anaesthesia available at that time.

After lunch we gathered in theatre to witness the resolution of the enigma. The old fellow, greatly impressed by the coterie of top brass gathered on his account, had been made as comfortable as possible on the operating table. Green drapes from neck to toe covered his body leaving the side of his right chest exposed to our anticipatory gaze. A purple mark with an indelible pencil identified the level of the ninth rib and the position of the incision. Armed with a syringe full of local anaesthetic Crikey began a series of injections accompanied by a non-stop flow of casual patter that surprised us all - our boss was normally committed to short sentences and long silences.

His elderly patient, successfully distracted, responded with his contribution of trivia and within minutes the skin was anaesthetised and incised exposing a few inches of the crucial ninth rib. Two snips with the rib shears (gardener's secateurs would have made a good substitute) released a section of the bone. The thin layer of tissue that now lay between the surgeon and our mystery was incised sufficiently for Crikey to insert an exploratory finger.

Now surgeons are an interesting study when they have to concentrate exclusively on information gathered from the sensory nerve endings of a finger that is exploring a hidden space. Some stare ahead, focussed on the middle distance as they gather and interpret their harvest of tactile data. Others concentrate their gaze where the digit would be were it visible - at the same time willing transparency on the tissues that hide it. Yet others roll their eyes heavenwards as though in silent prayer, imploring divine intervention - a welcome ally in all cases of surgical doubt. Crikey tilted his head to one side in a gesture of attentive enquiry and contemplated the far corner of the theatre with silent intensity.

"Crikey!" he observed with a slight frown as he lowered his gaze to engage our expectant faces one at a time, thus ensuring complete attention. (The actor in every surgeon enjoys a little limelight.) A heavy silence gathered under the theatre light as the moment of truth approached. The only person in the room unaware of the unfolding drama was the patient. Overwhelmed by the influence of his pre-medication he was now asleep.

"Crikey" he repeated as he slowly withdrew his finger, hooked around a cyst the size of a grape and held it up in triumph.

"Hydatids!" we exclaimed in inspired unison.

Our sudden expression of enlightenment disturbed the dozing patient and he coughed, sending hundreds of identical cysts spewing from the incision. They bounced on the floor and then rolled randomly about the place to be crushed underfoot in a rude chorus of popping noises, as startled spectators stepped back. The theatre floor looked like a winery at the beginning of a grape harvest.

The sudden hubbub aroused the old chap. He took in the situation and began to laugh, sending thousands more cascading from the wound to dance and roll about the place. The more he observed the comical chaos erupting from his side the more he laughed until the cavity was empty and the storm subsided. The surgeon summed up the scene with one word - "Crikey."

A resourceful nurse on the periphery of the pantomime emerged, armed with a brush, shovel and bucket and began to gather up the extraordinary harvest, clearing a path to the feet of the surgeon and bringing the show to a close.

Our patient casually accepted the diagnosis of hydatids (after all most of his sheep were similarly affected). With his breathing capacity now greatly improved he remained forever grateful to Crikey who had not only given him a great tale to dine out on, but also the necessary breath with which to tell it.

WITCHCRAFT AND RINGS

Theatre Sisters are a conservative lot. They learn by experience that to throw out some item at the suggestion of one surgeon is to invite its demand by another. Consequently they err on the side of hoarding, in the reasonable expectation that sooner or later the object in question is likely to be called for again. In time their tidy, well stoked cupboards may include instruments and material that would not be out of place in a medical museum.

I was innocently nosing through the cabinets in theatre one day when I came upon a package bearing an ornate, turn-of-the-century label that declared the contents to be Sea-Tangle Tents. Here was practical witchcraft indeed - dried stalks of seaweed. Sea-Tangle seaweed has stalks that range from the thickness of your little finger to the diameter of your thumb. Once dried they shrink to about one fifth of their original size. When inserted into the cervix (mouth of the womb) they absorb moisture from the surrounding tissue and slowly expand, gently dilating the passage and can eventually lead to an abortion. They have been used since the late fourteenth century so we really did have some ancient technology here.

The fifties saw the heyday of the magical Graffenberg ring. Herr Graffenberg had a bright idea. He took some biologically inert gold wire - about as thick as domestic fuse wire - and wound it in a close spiral with an internal diameter that would just admit a match stick. He then bent his tiny spring into a circle and soldered the ends together.

Appropriately the final product looked for all the world like a wedding ring - but a ring that was easily distorted and able to return to its original shape afterwards. This device could be pushed through the cervix and into the womb of women who had already given birth. Here it would act as an irritant that usually discouraged further pregnancies from taking up residence.

It was, however, very difficult to insert the ring through the tight, narrow cervical canal of women who had never borne children. A significant disadvantage lay in the need for a general anaesthetic to remove it and many women carried their internal wedding ring through menopause and eventually to their graves.

In its day the Graffenberg ring certainly contributed to a lowered birth rate but occasional pregnancies did tarnish its image. Apocryphal stories of babies emerging clutching the ring in their tiny hands were based more on propaganda than physiology. By the early sixties the 'pill' would displace the ring as a contraceptive option and the demand for 'ring x-rays', just to confirm their presence and position, became a thing of the past.

Not all G.P.s were adept at inserting Graffenberg's contribution to birth control and in one case the ring became imbedded in the wall of the cervix instead of ending up in the cavity of the uterus. In the process of this misplacement, the soldered joint that held it in a circle was broken, so that the end of the spring projected menacingly back into the vagina.

The referral note from the G.P. said it all.

"Thank you for admitting Mrs. .... who has a broken Graffenberg ring embedded in her cervix. The sharp wire projecting from it is performing a contraceptive service beyond the parameters of the original design. Her husband is demanding its urgent removal."

One gathers grateful patients in a variety of ways.

FROM THE LAND OF THISTLES AND HAGGIS

One of the many pleasures associated with work in a country hospital is the link between hospital practice and care in the community, forged by the regular visits of the G.P.s to the institution - and so it was in Whangarei. Indeed, as most of our General Practitioners had worked there as House Surgeons, before hanging up their shingles in the town, it was quite natural for them to maintain contact. Not only did they know where morning and afternoon tea was served, they also knew the most rewarding times to attend. Fresh baked scones every Saturday morning.

To supplement the supply of home-grown graduates, New Zealand was actively encouraging doctors from the Commonwealth to practice here. This policy attracted many from the U.K. and South Africa. The former chose Northland in the mistaken belief that they would find a sub-tropical paradise and the latter did so to avoid the chilly climate further south. Whangarei won on both counts and thereby gained a wider range of accents.

Dr. Marshall, fresh from the cool mists of Scotland, dispensed the spoken music of his birthplace with every syllable he uttered. New to the town and its ways, he found himself rostered on as the G.P. on weekend call before he had had time to unpack his sporran. One house-call was to a woman in early labour. To announce her imminent arrival at the Maternity Annex and at the same time introduce himself to the staff there, he rang the unit and found himself addressing the Matron - a very competent lady who shared with her peers the view that doctors were really excess to requirement in her domain and the quicker they understood this the better. Merely admitting to being a doctor could precipitate a significant frosting of the atmosphere.

"Yes - Maternity."

"Och aye - its Doctor Marshall heere."

"And *who are you*?" She snapped.

"Och - I'm feen thanks - and hoo are you?"

It took a long time to assure Matt that he had not been singled out for special treatment, but it must have dampened his enthusiasm for obstetrics for a while. In later years he carved out a significant niche for himself in Sports Medicine.

Another Scot had taken up practice in Waipu, then nearly an hours drive to the south of Whangarei. Dr. McBirney found this Nova Scotian farming enclave very much to his liking and was accepted enthusiastically by the community he served as the their solo G.P. After a period living in a small rented house, he announced, with regret, that he would not be staying on. Suitable houses to rent were simply non-existent in this small, stable, farming community and the income from the practice did not give him the confidence to build his own home.

The locals received this news with alarm and responded with the single minded spirit that had sustained their forebears throughout the daunting journey from Nova Scotia and had continued to motivate them long after they had settled in Waipu.

A spokesman for the community was appointed to discuss the situation with the good doctor and in particular to determine where he would like to live, if he had the choice. Dr. McBirney innocently indicated the hills just to the north of the town which commanded a glorious view of Bream Bay and the Pacific Ocean beyond.

A posse was immediately dispatched in their Land Rovers to seek the preferred view and to identify those farmers who owned property relevant to their quest. With typical expedition a site was chosen, land was subdivided and a substantial house built. Dr. McBirney stayed on.

Although I had spoken to him many times on the phone during my two years as a house surgeon, I only met the man face to face on one occasion - and did not realise at the time I had done so.

It went like this. He rang one night, anxious to warn me that he was sending in a 'burst appendix' and advised me to prepare for theatre immediately. I asked about the history of the case and learned that the patient had had a continuous right sided bellyache all day and it was now pretty bad. Although this could well be early appendicitis it didn't sound like a burst appendix to me and I said as much. (True, such cases begin with the usual pain associated with appendicitis but it takes a lot longer than a day for the organ to reach the point of rupture and when it does the pain dramatically subsides for an hour or two and is then replaced by the overwhelming generalised abdominal pain of peritonitis.)

"Laddie" - there was a rough edge to his voice. "If this is nae a burst appendix I'll gee ye a bottle of whisky."

The patient did have early appendicitis and we took him to theatre that night. When he was discharged I wrote the usual letter to the G.P. outlining the patient's stay in the hospital and carefully avoided any reference to ruptured organs.

The incident was long forgotten, when late one wet winter evening I was approached in the darkened hospital corridor by a sinister figure encased in a dripping raincoat - collar turned up and hat pulled down like a character in a 'B' grade movie.

"Dee ye ken a Doctor Parkes?"

"Aye - I ken a Doctor Parkes"

"Gi the bastard this"

He thrust a brown paper parcel into my hands, spun on his heels and melted into the night.

It was a lovely drop and I wrote and told him so.

Despite (or perhaps because of) the generosity and support of the community, Dr. McBirney was trapped in a solo rural practice where time off becomes a guilt trip, home visits involve many hours of driving over rough country roads and being on call is a perpetual mill stone.

Not surprisingly the burden of duty, endlessly performed, took its toll. He died suddenly of a massive heart attack while on his rounds.

DICTATION AND BLOTTERS

Physicians play mental chess all day with symptoms and signs - they are in the problem solving business. Surgeons tend to inhabit the hands-on, fix-it world and are less inclined to bother with cryptic crosswords.

Clive Garlick was our Physician and like Clive Lambert (whom he would soon replace as Superintendent when Crikey lost his battle with cancer) had also spent his early professional years in country hospitals while he studied for his post graduate qualifications - in itself quite a feat of acaedemic achievement. His duties included regular visits to the remote small hospitals scattered around Northland, as did other specialists who served at Whangarei.

The post-war decade saw many technological innovations gradually creep into common usage - some even reached rural hospitals. One such novelty was the small, reel-to-reel dictaphone. After years of writing out letters in longhand with a fountain pen and then handing them on for typing, the senior medical staff could now borrow the firm's dictaphone.

One of the first letters composed in this way involved a patient suffering from intermittent claudication and the letter to the referring G.P. should have read -

'Thank you for referring your patient complaining of intermittent claudication.'

Now 'claudication' comes from the Latin word meaning 'to limp' and in this case the limping is caused by poor circulation in the legs. Sufferers must pause at regular intervals to allow the blood supply in the legs to catch up with the demand and thus ease the cramping pain.

The letter came back from the typist -

'Thank you for referring your patient complaining of intermittent fornication.'

Articulation and enunciation became important elements in dictation thereafter.

It was in the fifties that the pharmaceutical industry began communicating directly with doctors, either through the mail or by personal representation, distributing modest tokens as reminders of their products. In the pre-biro days the Parker fountain pen ruled in professional circles and blotting paper, carrying on one side a message from the company, became the universal promoter of brand names. Every doctor had a drawer full of blotters.

When Dr. Garlick's children announced that they were due to begin using pen and ink at school and could they please have some blotting paper to take along, he saw a welcome opportunity to empty a drawer or two in his office. Lucky his wife had the good sense to censor the pile of blotters on offer before their redistribution among the innocents. A great many of them promoted pharmaceuticals dedicated to female hygiene - complete with illustrations. These juveniles may have been ready for the grown-up application of ink, but they were certainly not prepared for the adult advice that decorated some blotting paper.

TB - A SENTENCE

Pulmonary tuberculosis, that barometer of community well being, was a major health problem by mid 20th Century. Two world wars separated by a world depression had laid the poverty foundations for a pandemic that included New Zealand. Drugs that could theoretically eliminate the disease - when supported by good nutrition and adequate rest - became available in the late forties and for the first time in human history the tide began to turn. Patients diagnosed early enough could be almost guaranteed a cure at last. The problem now was to stop the further spread of the disease from the sufferer to the healthy individual. There were two main links that had to be broken. Because dairy cows were often infected, all raw milk had to be sterilised either by boiling in the kitchen or by pasteurisation at the factory - and all human cases that had the bacilli in their sputum had to be compulsorily isolated (through an act of Parliament) from the rest of society until their sputum was consistently clear of the causative organism and they could be legally declared 'non infectious'.

Patients deemed to be infectious were imprisoned in the T.B. Shelters - isolated hospital wards where treatment was compulsory and where progress could be monitored through regular chest x-rays and sputum analysis. In the days before effective medication this isolation was measured in years, but it was now down to six months for early cases. Maori were once again over-represented in T.B. statistics.

The impact of the anti-tuberculosis drugs was sufficiently dramatic to raise the reasonable expectation that this disease could eventually be eradicated from our shores. The success of early treatment raised public confidence in the programme and the value of early detection eventually became acceptable to the individual. Mobile x-ray units constantly toured the country in search of new cases and the public responded positively to the prospect of free chest x-rays. These 'T.B. Caravans' made regular appearances at most outdoor public gatherings.

This war was seen as winnable and although the nation's T.B. Shelters were still full at the end of the 1950's, we were only a decade away from closing most of them, and many Chest Physicians would see their speciality as 'T.B. doctors' evaporate in the apparent victory of Public Health policy.

Sterling stuff indeed. For the thirty years that followed, tuberculosis would remain a Third World disease, rarely diagnosed in New Zealand - and even then the patient would usually be a new arrival in the country. A major battle had been won but the war was not over. In the last decade of the Twentieth Century, as a reflection of new-found poverty, the bacillus was spreading once more. Over crowding and poor housing have recently conspired to re-ignite old fires.

Today a dark cloud is gathering over Russia where an epidemic of T.B. has erupted among the prison population. Here, inadequate drug treatment has led to the emergence of a strain of the bacillus that is resistant to all anti-tuberculous drugs. This T.B. super bug can drag us back into the Dark Ages and in the process wipe out the progress achieved in the past half century.

In Whangarei our Chest Physician was Dr. Adrian Webb, a gentleman of the old school with a passion for theatre and opera that was so intense it could induce him to drive to Auckland on regular occasions just to take in a show.

Adrian was one of many T.B. specialists who had studied their subject while incarcerated in a T.B. shelter as a patient. Because of this experience he had a special empathy with his patients - which they reciprocated. His responsibilities included an overview of all T.B. cases in the province and involved links with the Health Department as well. His long term goal was to work himself out of a job - and he succeeded.

Whangarei's purpose built T.B. Shelter consisted of a men's and a women's ward and a nursing station. Windows everywhere admitted both the healing sunlight and beneficial fresh air. A glass house with tempting views of the forbidden outside world.

Spouses could visit provided they maintained a discrete distance, but children were restricted to peering in at their parent from outside the transparent glass prison. A remarkable number of marriages survived this unexpected and indefinitely extendable challenge - many others failed.

Each town had an active 'T.B. Association' which struggled to support families as they picked their way through the social and financial wilderness that engulfed them on the day a family member was declared to have a 'positive spit'. The whole policy of T.B. management was firmly based on the greatest good for the greatest number. Individual rights - by consensus - became subjugated under the 'Infectious Diseases Act'.

Boredom, complicated by inactivity and imposed under the banner of 'rest' as the cornerstone of management, was the patient's daily burden. It was in T.B. shelters that the profession of Occupational Therapy found early fertile ground as it supervised the production of literally thousands of wicker baskets and fluffy teddy bears.

Although daytime dragged itself out at the pace of a reluctant snail, the patient's nights were usually sweet and gentle events. Each evening a generous dose of Linctus Heronii (a derivative of morphine) was served up to suppress the familiar daytime chorus of brassy coughing and eased the patient into the comforting arm of Morpheus - the Roman god of dreams.

One dreaded complication of pulmonary tuberculosis was the development of an abscess of the lungs. This would arise when the disease had rotted out a cavity ranging in size from a walnut to a small orange, in one or both lungs - usually near the top. The resultant ragged hole was always loath to close and ever ready to expand. Eventually when anaesthetists had mastered the art of rhymically pumping gasses into the lungs instead of relying on the patient's own respiratory efforts to maintain breathing, chest surgeons would solve the problem by excising the offending lung segment. However for Whangarei this solution was still a few years away.

Instead we continued to hang our faith on compressing the lung and thereby eventually obliterating the cavity. In some cases segments of several adjacent ribs would be removed without entering the thoratic cavity, thus allowing the chest wall to sag inwards and squeeze the lung. Other patients lay about on beds for hours with their chests loaded with small sand bags heaped on the appropriate side in an attempt to compress the lesion.

Eventually someone, somewhere, had the bright idea of squeezing the lung by pumping a measured quantity of air into the thoracic space that surrounds each lung. This manoeuvre was the most effective measure to date and I came onto the scene after this had become standard practice.

The business of pumping air into the thoracic space was fine where only one lung was involved in the cavitation process. In cases where both lungs were diseased it was safer to pump air into the abdominal cavity, thus pushing the diaphragm upwards and modestly compressing both thoracic spaces without hampering normal breathing. Over a period of a couple of weeks this air would be absorbed and the process would have to be repeated regularly for a few months.

It fell upon the shoulders of the house surgeon to introduce a needle into the appropriate space and using a beautiful, shiny brass pump, housed in a varnished mahogany box, pump the prescribed volume of air into the patient. The trick was to get the needle into the correct place without perforating either the lung in one case or the bowel in the other. The whole business proceeded by feel alone. One first experienced the sudden 'give' as the resistance of the skin was overcome followed by the easier passage through the softness of the muscle, culminating in the distinctive 'pop' as the needle finally passed through the inner lining. Given this tactile sequence one would be confident of the correct placement and proceed with the pumping.

Occasionally the anti-tuberculous drugs had rendered the sputum negative by this stage in the disease and the management of many lung cavities could proceed on an outpatient basis. At regular intervals such patients would report to the unit for a progress chest x-ray and a top-up of free air. I was busy with the little brass pump one morning when George turned up for some more air in his belly. As soon as this had been completed he rushed away without the exchange of chit-chat that his visits usually involved.

"George is in a bit of a scurry today," I remarked to the nurse.

"Yes - it's high tide at two o'clock," she replied.

It transpired that George had a summer party trick that he was anxious to repeat. With a tummy full of air he would hurry home to don his swimming gear and wade out into the deep water surrounded by unsuspecting fellow swimmers until his feet left the bottom. At this stage the water would be part way up his chest, but the additional abdominal air rendered him buoyant while still vertical. He would then 'walk' out to the channel marker while treading water, surrounded by incredulous bathers. I guess when your world was clouded by T.B. you caught your fun where you could.

CHILD STRAIGHTENERS

Once upon a time Orthopaedic Surgeons were gentle fellows. Their speciality was born when the smoke and smog generated by the Industrial Revolution had effectively blocked out the sunlight that was responsible for the production of vitamin D in the skin of growing children. This vitamin lack inhibited their bone maturation, resulting in a condition known as rickets, where the leg bones bowed under the weight of the growing body. Doctors who specialised in straightening these young limbs turned to the Greek language for a name. They combined the word 'orthos' (meaning straight) with 'paideia' (rearing children), giving them 'orthopaedic' - child straighteners.

The same Industrial Revolution that gave the ultraviolet inhibiting, smoky atmosphere of the 'Black Country' also created heavy industry and the increased trauma to workers that came with it. Our child straighteners, with their interest in bones and joints, moved into dealing with smashed up adults and in the process hyjacked the limb amputation market from the General Surgeons. As part of this transition they needed to find the self assurance and autocratic manner that would enable them to make shattering decisions regarding which patients could or could not retain a full complement of limbs. A far cry from gently straightening out bent kids. Thus a new breed of surgeons was born.

This dogmatic self confidence became the hallmark of their calling until the post-war antibiotic era enabled a more conservative approach to bone trauma, now freed from the haunting fears of gangrene and blood poisoning. Limbs were more likely to be saved than amputated and with this change came a welcome mellowing of the stereotype.

Whangarei's first Orthopaedic Surgeon, Fred Gruar, had inherited something of the old manner from his tutors - and it often showed. However, the odd ranting tantrum was offset by his undoubted technical skill and sound judgement.

All house surgeons initially feared him - all nurses were perpetually terrified of him and most of his patients loved him this side of idolatry. Colourful characters are one thing - Fred came in glorious technicolour.

I successfully avoided direct contact with Fred throughout my first six months in Whangarei. There was, however, no permanent escape. I eventually had to do the orthopaedic run.

It all began in the Outpatient Clinic. Fred ushered me into a cubicle occupied by a young teenaged boy and his mother.

"What's wrong with him?" he snarled - and left me to it.

The lad had an acutely tender spot just below his kneecap. It had been a problem for some weeks and there was no history of injury. I hadn't the faintest idea what it was all about and told Fred as much upon his return.

He, in turn, exploded.

"Are you going to be the sort of doctor who can't explain a simple lesion like this? His mother wants to know all about her son's knee - she wants to know if it needs an operation - will he be crippled? Are you going to be the sort of G.P. who sends everything to outpatients?"

Turning to the mother he snarled -

"It's Osgood Schlatters Disease" and stalked away.

I was terrified to hear myself shouting after him -

"That's told the mother a fat lot!"

His long white coat described a graceful arc as he spun around and roared with laughter.

"You're right you know, " and returned to give all three of us an erudite dissertation on the condition - its history, origin and prognosis, including the reassuring observation that most cases clear up spontaneously in a matter of months.

From that moment on Fred and I were friends and what is more, I now had a clear understanding of this form of osteochondritis. I was supremely confident of recognising the next one when it turned up. In forty years I never saw another example.

Hereafter, Fred was a delight to work for. In theatre he explained everything as he progressed through the operation and was always willing to allow me to take an active part in the procedure. I loved it.

However he did have an annoying habit of involving the theatre nursing staff in his cross examinations, expecting them to have the same level of knowledge as he would a colleague. One of his favourite questions used to be -

"Why am I doing this operation nurse?"

He was stopped in his tracks one day when a particularly bright young lady replied - "I expect you need the practice - Sir."

His laughter at this response eased the tension and this particular pointless question was put to rest for a long time.

Many Orthopaedic Surgeons added poliomyelitis to their quiver of interests when epidemics of this viral disease flared up around the world. In the late thirties, when I was at primary school, an outbreak spread throughout New Zealand mainly effecting school children. This predilection to attack the young gave it the popular name of 'Infantile Paralysis.' A causative factor was believed to be exposure of the neck to the rays of summer sunshine. As a protective manoeuvre kids were decked out in sun hats with a flap hanging down from the back of the hat to shade their necks. This novel headwear was readily accepted by school children because of its exciting association with the hats worn by members of the French Foreign Legion and popularised by the adventures of Beau Geste. The wheel of fashion has now turned full circle. Today we deck out our children in similar head gear to protect them from the evils of rampant ultraviolet light.

'Infantile Paralysis' became 'Poliomyelitis' when the disease returned a decade later, attacking young adults. This time it lingered in the community, slowly extending its effects over a wider spectrum of age groups throughout the 1950's.

The possibility that any sudden weakness of a young limb could be a manifestation of polio was foremost in most doctor's minds at this time. Fred was quick to recognise this possibility when a couple, who were friends of his, rang him about their child. On the strength of their story Fred urged the parents to meet him at the Children's Ward immediately.

The toddler was a bright wee thing who had only recently mastered the complex business of walking, but now, repeated attempts to place the child in the standing position, resulted in the immediate buckling of his right leg - indicating that it was too weak to support the child's weight. The diagnosis was obvious.

While Sister Abbott (known affectionately as 'Bud') took the child away to admit him to the ward, Fred, with gentleness and compassion, outlined the gloomy prognosis for a child so young afflicted with polio. The parents were devastated and reacted accordingly.

I arrived at the peak of this tearful consultation, feeling like a fish out of water, in the midst of the sobbing. I looked up when Bud appeared at the office doorway. She was smiling ever so sweetly with a toddler standing beside her, eager to break away and totter over to his grieving mother.

While Bud was changing the child into regulation pyjamas, she noted a small sliver of glass embedded in the child's right foot and promptly removed it with miraculous results. Fred dined out on this tale for years.

NAILS, SCREWS AND BONES

When Allied prisoners of war were released from Germany at the end of World War Two, British orthopaedic surgeons were amazed at the treatment given fractured femurs by their German colleagues. Fractured thigh bones were a common war injury and in those days would be treated with bed rest and traction for many weeks. Instead the Germans had operated on them, driving a long 'nail' down the entire length of the marrow cavity, thus internally splinting the fractured bone. Within a few days the patient could be mobilised.

After the war the rest of the world eagerly caught up with this radical step in orthopaedic surgery and metallic internal splinting was vigorously explored. The various metal devices employed in this new approach carried the German names of their inventors so that a catalogue of orthopaedic equipment began to look like a section from a Berlin phone book. Orthopaedic surgeons now assumed the mantle of engineers and became preoccupied with the pitch of screw threads and the tensile strength of alloys. Out of this eventually evolved the ubiquitous (and profitable) modern hip replacement.

In the first post-war decade, the prosthetic techniques of orthopaedics had taken root in New Zealand. Fred had been keen to keep up with each new development and made frequent journeys to Auckland for this purpose. After one such trip he returned all fired up with a new approach to the painful osteoarthritic hip joint. In this condition both of the bone surfaces involved in the joint have become roughened. Pain would be generated when these two rough surfaces ground against each other with every movement.

The new management solution involved opening up the joint, dislocating it so that the diseased round knob at the end of the bone could be exposed and sawn off. A smooth metal facsimile of the round head of the femur, mounted on a long metal pin (not unlike a giant drawing pin) could then be used to replace the discarded bone. The long spike attached to the underside of the metal knob could then be driven down the marrow cavity of the femoral neck to firmly attach the prosthesis. This done, the dislocated joint could be restored to its proper place and the wound closed.

When repeating this operation, following a demonstration in Auckland a few weeks earlier, Fred ran into trouble. As he twisted the leg in order to dislocate the joint, he managed to fracture the shaft of the femur instead (old bones are notoriously brittle). Now he had to internally splint the broken bone as well as perform the planned procedure.

He was both embarrassed and annoyed at the same time and when the extended performance was finally completed he gave orders that he be notified the minute the patient showed the first signs of recovery from the anaesthetic.

In due course the awaited message was delivered and Fred stormed into the recovery cubicle in the ward and shouted into the ear of the restless, awakening patient -

"Why didn't you tell me you had soft bones!"

The information must have satisfactorily penetrated into the depths of the slowly clearing brain because the patient apologised to everyone - including Fred - for her failure to realise the fragile state of her ageing skeleton, assuring all and sundry that had she only known she would certainly have shared such knowledge with her surgeon.

The word 'litigation' had not yet entered the vocabulary of our patients.

When old folk fall over they often suffer hip fractures and these, in the past, like fractures of the thigh, could only be treated by bed rest and traction extending over several weeks. During this period of enforced inactivity the elderly patient was at great risk of bed sores and fatal pneumonia. Internal fixation of such fractures greatly reduced both mortality and morbidity and had the patient home in less than half the time.

Now, the femur is an odd shaped bone. It consists of a long shaft that runs up from the knee to the level of the hip joint. At this point it gives off a 'neck' a few centimetres long that runs inwards and upwards to end in a knob the size of a golf ball. It is this golf ball (the femoral head) that lies in a shallow saucer shaped depression in the pelvis to form the hip joint. Fractures of the hip are usually fractures of the neck part - often at the level that the neck joins the rounded head.

By drilling a hole through the top of the shaft opposite the point where the neck emerges, it is possible to drive a fluted nail up the marrow cavity of the neck and impact the end of the nail into the golf ball head - thus bridging the fracture and splinting it internally. The head of the nail can now be secured to the shaft of the femur to strengthen the arrangement. It is wonderful what you can do with a meccano set.

I had assisted Fred with one of these hip pinning operations just before the Christmas holidays that found me on duty and Fred an hour's drive up the coast at Oakura relaxing in the sun.

On Boxing Day I admitted an elderly Scottish lady who had fallen while touring Northland and had sustained a fractured hip - one that was ideal for pinning.

When on holiday at Oakura, Fred could be contacted for advice or called back on duty by leaving a message at the beach store, which had one of the few telephones in the area. Each morning at ten he would call at the shop for supplies and respond to any appeals for guidance. I had left a message for him earlier in the morning and he obligingly rang back.

I told him of our new case.

"Is she fit?"

"Yes."

"Then pin the bastard" - and he hung up.

I was in the staffroom when he called and I turned to Bob Mulligan, the duty general surgeon, with the news.

"Have you ever seen one done?" he asked.

"One," I replied.

"Well that's one more than me - but I'll come for moral support if you like."

"Thanks Bob."

I have since discovered that the first time you fly solo with an operation it goes like a charm - it is on subsequent occasions that everything turns to custard. This event was no exception - much to the relief of Bob, the theatre and x-ray staff and myself.

A week later Fred was back from holiday and making his first ward round.

"Who's in the side room?"

"The Scottish lady with the neck of femur - the one I rang you about."

"How's she doing?"

"Ok."

"Let's see." And clutching an envelope crammed with the relevant x-rays he led us to the bedside.

"Good morning - I'm Mr. Gruar. What part of Scotland are you from?"

"Edinburgh."

"Indeed. I studied orthopaedics there."

"Is that so young man - well in that case perhaps you will show me the skiagraphs?"

'Skiagraph' is an old fashioned name for x-ray images (literally 'shadow pictures') and her choice of this word made Fred a little uneasy.

"Oh - I doubt you would understand them," he countered vaguely.

"Mebe" she responded.

"Mebe ye ken my brother. He is Professor of Orthopaedics at Edinburgh University."

"Oh - in that case." Fred withdrew the films from the envelope with a slightly shaking hand.

"Now you can see here where I inserted the guide wires for the nail. I chose this one to guide the nail - see how it points directly to the centre of the head - now this one shows how I attached the plate......"

He went on to assure her that all was well - a text book case - she should be up and about as soon as the sutures were removed.

So saying he backed away from the near royal presence and the room was evacuated with almost indecent haste.

Once safely outside and beyond earshot he turned to me and in a stage whisper he snarled - "If she ever finds out *you* did it I'll kill ya!"

HOKIANGA

BEYOND THE BLACK STUMP

At the end of our first year as house surgeons we could at last apply for full registration and thus gain the right to practice medicine unsupervised. Some of our number eagerly took the opportunity to enter the lucrative field of general practice, but most of us stayed on, either to gain more experience or to prepare for later specialisation. I chose to remain in hospital practice but had no intention of sitting further examinations.

It was about half way through the second year that Crikey Lambert found me drinking coffee in the staff room and solemnly invited me into his office.

It transpired that on the previous evening the Superintendent of Rawene Hospital (about three hours drive to the north and west of Whangarei) had dropped dead. He felt that it was imperative that a replacement arrive the next day and had decided to send me. Any questions? A word that I dared not utter flickered at the back of my mind - 'crikey'.

Next morning I was packed and driving north in search of the Hokianga, guided by the invaluable system of black on yellow A.A. signs. Only short stretches of the road sported tar seal and these islands of motoring luxury became more abbreviated as the journey continued. The north road was reasonably wide and well maintained, but each westward turn-off offered a distinct decline in travelling comfort. There could be little doubt that I was now heading way beyond the black stump.

With the deterioration of the carriage-way came a change in the roadside scene. Shrouded, bush-clad hills rose higher and crowded the diminishing pasture. Houses became smaller and spoke of poverty and neglect. That tell-tale of farming prosperity - the roadside fence - staggered along unevenly, struggling to contain the margins of the property like the remnants of a shattered army limping along in single file.

I was just inside the boundary of the Hokianga County and passing through the tiny settlement of Waima when it first happened. A chap on the roadside acknowledged my passing with a casual nod of recognition.

"Wrong bloke - you don't know me" I muttered as I left him enveloped in my swirling dust trail. An oncoming motorist - the first in many miles - raised a hand from the steering wheel in relaxed salutation as we rattled past each other. Further on, some kids sitting on a cream stand waved enthusiastically at my approach. Emboldened I waved back - this was a game anyone could play. I got in early as I approached the next stranger and gave him an acknowledging nod which was instantly returned. And so it continued as the road narrowed, the pot holes deepened and the town of Rawene drew closer.

This was the Hokianga, where everyone acknowledged the existence of everyone else in a spirit of mutual interdependence. Merely by being there you were part of it and graciously accepted without question. I was experiencing the essence of the place even before my feet had touched its soil. Initiation was completed with a nod, a smile or a wave. I don't have to know you to acknowledge your presence, but having done so we are no longer strangers. Now there is a welcome for you.

From the Waima saddle the road descends, winding along the mangrove trimmed margin of the upper harbour before heading towards a hill capped by rambling wooden buildings punctuated by a water tower and an erect boiler-house chimney. This had to be the hospital, raised above the unhealthy morning mists and overlooking the town beyond. As an expression of inspired forward planning - and for greater user convenience - the cemetery lay opposite.

Through their glorious panoramic view of the surrounding countryside, including the harbour and the road, the hospital staff had observed my approach and had a small welcoming committee in place at the main entrance anticipating my arrival. In those days, merely to own a second hand car was an inflated status symbol and a new vehicle required access to overseas funds - not a common feature in the Hokianga. Everyone could be identified by the car they drove and strangers were obvious a mile away.

I was about to meet a remarkable woman - Matron Renee Shadbolt. She was easily the tallest and occupied the centre of the group framed by the doorway. Her uniform had the 'slept-in' look and her matron's veil drooped in defiance of starchy conventional expectations. Stepping forward she extended her hand -

"Welcome *doctor*" she announced emphasising the second word with a hint of challenge in her voice.

I guessed her to be my senior by about twenty years and realised immediately that in the circumstances I needed her more than she needed me - and adapted my manner accordingly.

A decade had passed since the legendary Dr. G.M. Smith had left the district after thirty-four years of service and during those ten years as many doctors had come and gone. The one constant presence during that unstable period had been Renee and now another transient was on her door step. Doctors were ten-a-penny in her world.

After lunch she took me on a tour of her hospital. As a medical student I had read some of the books written by the outspoken father of the Hokianga Special Area and from them had gained a healthy respect for G.M. Smith. Indeed this influence had drawn me north after graduation. However I had not expected to work so soon so close to his shadow. Above the door to the consulting room a photo of GM glowered down on the waiting room - a bird's nest of tangled hair and a pipe gripped determinedly between clenched teeth, defying anyone to challenge his authority. They must have been heady days for the Hokianga.

The hospital had been built to his design and very much under his critical supervision. From the ceiling of every corridor a spaghetti of pipes carrying steam, water, power and telephone lines was suspended in unsightly confusion. The aesthetics of this arrangement was constantly questioned but the maintenance workers appreciated its glorious simplicity and accessibility. Leaking water and steam pipes could be quickly identified and readily repaired. His provision of isolated rooms where all wound dressings were undertaken was a vast improvement on the old practice of attending to such matters within the open ward with the consequent risk of cross infection.

We had completed the tour and I was preparing to drive down to the Rawene Pub (which was to be my home until the Superintendent's house had been cleared for my use) when Renee accosted me with the news that we had trouble looming in the Maternity Unit. Now, Renee had a curious tic that involved rapid, involuntary blinking. The more relaxed she was the more her eyelids fluttered over cool steel-blue eyes. When she was under pressure the eyelids seemed to tense and the tic would disappear, suddenly exposing everyone to her steady, icy gaze.

I froze under her gaze, like a rabbit caught in headlights, as she outlined the situation. Given the circumstances it was clear that assistance with obstetric forceps was indicated. I was thrown a little when Renee offered to give the anaesthetic while I wrestled with the forceps.

The risk of disaster here lay in the anaesthetic and I had a sudden image of myself standing in a Coroner's Court, hand on the Bible, desperately trying to explain why I chose to allow a person 'other than a duly registered and qualified Medical Practitioner' to administer an anaesthetic while I, who had no significant experience with forceps, had complicated the undertaking by prolonging the endeavour.

The implied challenge of the formal welcome now resurfaced and required immediate resolution.

"Look, you have had vastly more experience with forceps than I have - how about I give the dope and you handle the tongs?"

Her face relaxed with this proposition and the comforting blink returned, endorsing approval.

The mother was soon anaesthetised and with obvious pride in her skill, Renee presented the world with yet another live babe to her credit - and I made a friend through mutual respect.

It was late afternoon before I was free to drive down to the pub - casually exchanging nods and waves with pedestrians - like a royal tour in slow motion.

The foyer was deserted and I found the publican serving a modest sprinkling of patrons in the public bar.

"You'll be the new doctor" he volunteered in greeting. "Staying long?"

"I'm only here for a while - until a new appointment can be made."

"Me too - I came here to relieve for a month - that was twelve years ago. This here's Jack." he added, indicating a middle aged man leaning on the bar. "He came five years ago as a temporary clerk."

A tall young man rose from the window seat that commanded a view of the street and walked over with outstretched hand.

"I'm Shane the chemist - welcome to the back of beyond. Be staying long?"

"Er - not sure really," I mumbled, recalling the earlier conversation.

"Bring your drink over to the window - I need to keep an eye on the shop. Trade is really quiet in the mornings - but it eases up a lot in the afternoons."

We chatted on as he watched his shop door across the road - ever ready to slip back to his business at the first sign of a customer.

The phone on the wall gave two short rings and fell silent. Despite an obviously aborted call the barman, to my surprise, ambled over to the instrument, raised the receiver and answered it. I had failed to recognise that I was now in the world of manual telephones and party lines where Morse Code ruled.

"It's for you," he announced, waving the receiver towards me.

Crikey was on the other end and I felt slightly guilty to have my boss ring me at a public bar. His usual brief conversations were even further abbreviated when conveyed by toll call. I gathered that relief was already on its way in the form of a G.P. and I was to stay for at least a week while the new chap settled in and then report back.

The Hokianga Special Area (of which I was now temporary director) boasted two medical appointments in Rawene - a Hospital Superintendent (and director) supported by a G.P. in the town. This latter post had fallen vacant some weeks previously and it was the sudden death of the superintendent that made my trip essential.

As well as Hospital Superintendent and temporary Director of the Special Area, I was also seconded as Port Health Officer and New Zealand Railways Medical Officer - yet, from my recent conversation with the boss it already looked as though my multiple temporary appointments could well be the shortest in Rawene's living memory.

Next morning I was the sole diner at breakfast when mine host hurried over and announced with obvious concern:-

"You owe me a girl!"

Now, among the many positions I temporarily occupied in this county, supplying women - for what ever purpose - was not one that readily sprang to mind.

"Oh - how come?"

"Well one of my cleaners left me this morning to work in your hospital so I need one of your girls to fill the gap. The only employers of casual staff in this town are you and me, so you owe me one - otherwise it gets out of balance."

"I'll see what I can do" I volunteered vaguely, without really understanding what I was talking about.

He was all smiles that evening when I returned.

"Thanks mate - she came down this afternoon after an argument with one of your supervisors - so we're quits."

I dismissed his expression of gratitude with a casual 'Think nothing of it' and silently looked forward to a period of calm in industrial relationships.

The Outpatient's Clinic that day had been an education. The Hospital telephonist cum Receptionist cum Medical Records Clerk had been seconded as my nurse cum chaperone.

The first case - a middle aged Maori woman, mentioned that she had been an inpatient a few months previously so I asked my multi talented helper for the old notes. She returned in triumph a few minutes later waving a single sheet of paper which turned out to be the temperature chart from the admission in question.

"Is that all?" I queried.

"It's all there" she replied defensively.

The single sheet bore the patient's name and the records of twice daily temperature, pulse and respiratory rate faithfully plotted for a period of six days.

Alongside the first day was written:-

"Admitted with breast abscess R."

The next day was annotated:-

"Abscess incised."

The succeeding two days bore the repeated inscription:-

"Discharging."

The fifth day announced.

"Discharge stopped."

And across the sixth day was written:-

"Discharged."

She was right - it was all there.

The clinic was completed by mid morning and my assistant adopted yet another role and made us both a cup of tea. It was during this period of civilised relaxation that an excited Renee swept into the room with eyes aflutter.

"Doctor - doctor - we have an emergency and this time *I* will give the anaesthetic and *you* can do the surgery."

It was the twinkle in those eyes that cautioned me to play along for the meantime at least.

"He's all ready for you *doctor*," she confided as she pushed open the dressing room door.

The examination couch was empty. A shamefaced boy about ten stood by the bedside locker gently patting his enormous black dog which sat on the locker top surveying me with doleful eyes that implored forgiveness. (Norman Rockwell would have loved it). Firmly embedded in the dog's lower lip was a fish hook.

Armed with a bottle of ether and a face cloth, Renee had that animal asleep in no time allowing me to demonstrate the consummate surgical skill needed to push the barb of the hook out through the lip and snip the shank off with a pair of pliers. I suspected that the dog had been secretly sedated by Renee prior to the undertaking - but did not ask.

A bloke, who had smashed up his leg in a tractor accident, came in an ambulance that afternoon and after an hours drive over Hokianga roads he was pretty distressed. While the staff were busy organising his admission I decided to get some pethidine into him. When I asked for the drug cupboard keys I was told I would not need them - just go into the ward office. So I did.

Fastened to the office wall was a locked wooden cabinet about the size of a modern microwave oven. On top of it was heaped, small, labelled, cardboard boxes containing the full range of dangerous drugs - omnopon - morphine - pethidine and enough barbiturates in various forms to sedate an entire zoo. I took what I wanted - noted it in the Dangerous Drugs Register that hung from a nail alongside - and returned to complete the task.

As soon as the patient was comfortable, I took the Duty Sister aside and casually enquired into the storage of dangerous drugs. She assured me that they had been on the top of the cupboard for as long as she could remember.

"You must realise doctor that nobody in the Hokianga is interested in that sort of stuff, so there really is no point in locking them away - anyway there isn't any room for them."

"Well what is inside the cabinet?"

"Aspros - safety pins - scissors and sticking plaster - they wouldn't last five minutes around here if they weren't safely under lock and key."

IN RESIDENCE

The Superintendent's house stood astride a ridge just below the hospital grounds. It was of recent construction and adequately appointed. To the west it looked down the harbour past a zig-zag of headlands and brooding hills; an ever changing prospect that reflected every whim of weather and nuance of light - yet the basic structure of this landscape had remained constant for centuries. A war canoe or a square rigged sailing ship, struggling against the tide, would still fit in perfectly.

On the eastern side the prospect involved a complex system of rivers and creeks flanked with mangroves and mudflats that would lie exposed twice daily. Here erosion and the consequent silting had taken its toll and told the tale of post-European deforestation leaving a scabby countryside slowly slipping into the sea. Early morning light would often play magician. Boggy mudflats, fleetingly encrusted with silver and curtained by patches of soft white mist, made mornings a delight.

I loved the place and moved in on the third day. My immediate needs were few and simple - and one of them was an electric iron. On my first evening in residence I packed my un-ironed laundry and took it up to the hospital to complete this domestic chore.

The prospect of a doctor ironing his shirts delighted both Renee and the rest of the audience that gathered each evening in the staff room. The priest was there together with half of the off-duty nursing staff and a few patients and relatives of patients that were still on the 'sick list'. Rawene was half a century ahead of today's hospitals that have only recently acknowledged the value of families sharing in the healing process. The Hokianga would always find a bed for anxious relatives. There they were - a ragtag cluster of carers watching the doctor iron his shirts.

I knew that Renee, in company with two other New Zealand nurses, had served in Spain during the Spanish Civil War and I gently prompted her to recall and share that adventure.

Her response was dramatic in every sense of the word. She treated us to an extremely animated, one-woman re-enactment of the experience. Her setpiece focussed on the Spanish wound dressers. Apparently men attended to this task over there and they felt threatened by foreign, female nurses. These dressers were very proud of their sparkling instruments, literally spitting on them and polishing their surfaces with dirty old rags at every opportunity. Renee and her companions, on the other hand, boiled their surgical hardware vigorously in the hard, limey water of the region to ensure sterility. Their tools of trade emerged from the boiling water sterile but dulled by a fine coating of lime.

With eyes a-flutter she pranced around the room miming the Spanish dresser's spit-and-polish approach and then, waving pretended forceps and scissors in front of imaginary patients, beseeched them to choose between their gleaming steel and the dirty, dull, surgical cutlery currently on offer by these alien women. The whole performance came wrapped in broken English and fractured Spanish. It was magnificent.

Her trip to Spain in support of the Anti-Facist cause had not endeared her to her government (indeed they almost managed to block it) - neither did the part she played following the 'Auckland riots' during the worst of the thirties depression.

She had been employed at Auckland Hospital when a rally of unemployed men held near the Town Hall, had suddenly spun out of control. It ended when every shop window in Queen Street had been broken and most of the contents looted.

Police and their supporters waged a long and bitter battle against the rioters, leaving many on both sides wounded. The Casualty department at Auckland Hospital was inundated with the injured who were promptly segregated into two groups according to the part they played. The firmly declared policy at the hospital was to leave the rioters (irrespective of the gravity of their wounds) until all others had been treated. The fact that the authorities (and in particular the medical staff) had endorsed this politically biased arrangement angered Renee and a small group of fellow nurses. They took over some clinic space and began treating the most seriously injured rioters - thereby incurring the censure of the hospital establishment for many years.

When I asked Renee about this episode in her life, her response was intense and chilling. The friendly flutter evaporated and her face and voice hardened as the recollection re-focussed. She found no humour in this event. It involved her people in her country and hinged on what she saw as the unforgivable sin of directing professional medical and nursing care according to arbitrarily perceived blame, ignoring the severity of humanitarian need. I was at once sorry that I had asked and yet glad to have learned more about this special woman.

ASSISTANCE ARRIVES

The news came through the next morning. The chap who had been appointed to the general practice position in the town, was on his way. He would set up home in G.M. Smith's old cottage in the valley below the hospital. A watch on the only road into Rawene was set up in the comfort of the hospital staff room and we settled back to wait.

"Here he comes" the lookout reported confidently and the doorstep welcoming committee casually took up their places. For me it was deja vu and having been initiated

I could now adopt a more detached role and drift off into the background.

A car pulled up - a figure emerged.

"Welcome *doctor*" - the subtle emphasis was there again and I knew that for the meantime he was on his own. There are times when being in the know can make one embarrassingly smug.

The hospital kept me busy while Renee and her team repeated the well rehearsed ritual of the grand tour and it was mid afternoon before I had time to visit our newcomer. I found him in the sitting room of his cottage surrounded by unopened cases.

The casual niceties that we employ when getting to know someone were quickly hijacked as he treated me to a flowing resume of his life and works to date, dwelling on his medical and surgical adventures in Tanganyika, Ethiopia, Kenya and a number of places I have never before heard of. Some quick mental arithmetic suggested he had already used up a couple of professional lifetimes in the ten years that made him my senior. As the flow of recollected achievements came to an end his brow furrowed -

"I say old chap - I have the most shocking migraine - do you think you could get me a hundred of pethidine - in an ampoule?"

Now I knew just where to go to satisfy this request - and did so - returning with the ampoule, a syringe and a swab of antiseptic-soaked cotton wool - all ready to give him an intra muscular injection.

He snatched up the glassware and with a display of sleight-of-hand that would have done credit to a seasoned conjurer, he cracked the ampoule - loaded the syringe - twisted his shirtsleeve into a tourniquet and unloaded the lot into a vein in his left arm.

"That was a hundred!" I gasped, expecting him to pass out any minute.

"Yeah - I know. Ah, that's better - thanks old chap." He began unpacking the nearest suitcase.

I gathered up the evidence and returned to the hospital where I rang Crikey *after* Renee and I had found somewhere safe to store the scissors, aspros, safety pins and sticking plaster and had placed the assorted narcotics securely under lock and key.

The irony was obvious. None of the staff, or public, had ever shown any interest in these drugs - it took a doctor to pose a threat. Of course it would have had to be done sooner or later - and this was a good wakeup call for everyone.

Crikey arrived the next morning. His approach was both unobserved and unannounced. In no time he had convinced the voluable new boy to seek treatment. Quite a feat for a man who rationed his sentences as tightly as the chief did.

Before they left the boss looked at me, shook his head slowly and said -

"Crikey - I think you'd better stay a bit longer."

So I did.

NURSES

In the Hokianga, nurses formed the backbone of the Special Area medical services and although the doctors involved did not always recognise this, the community was in no doubt about the nurse's place in the scheme of things.

The county is split into two halves by the sea, with Rawene well up harbour on the southern shore facing Kohukohu across the water. The two were linked by a passenger launch and a very basic 'vehicle' ferry in the form of a simple barge, pushed by a power boat.

It was kauri timber that first attracted Europeans to the district and as the bush was cleared, farming and erosion followed. In 1837 Baron de Thierry arrived from France via England intending to set himself up as "Sovereign Chief of New Zealand." Instead he sprinkled his noble gout genes about the place and left suddenly to become a music teacher in Auckland when Hone Heke got stroppy. A year later Bishop Pompallier turned up scattering Holy Water around and successfully established the Roman Catholic religion along the shores of the harbour.

The sea remained the principal link with the outside world until about sixty years ago when the Onehunga based coastal freighter "Hokianga" surrendered to road transport.

Roading that meandered between the various settlements on the Rawene side, was very poor and often impassable while the roads on the northern shore were considerably worse. A complicated timetable of launch routes criss-crossed the harbour for decades moving freight, people and cream in all weathers and all directions until the early fifties, when this service declined as the struggling land transport system slowly established its competitive edge.

Either way the communities dotted around the harbour existed in relative isolation one from the other and from the hospital facilities. Because of these restrictions on movement it made sense to station a nurse within most settlements, providing them with a house and a chain of small clinic buildings that they would attend regularly, with or without the support of a visiting doctor. Thus the nurse remained the primary focus for all manner of emergencies as well as for matters of continuing community and individual health. These nurses played a key part in the management of tuberculosis cases, controlling outbreaks of infectious diseases, in the provision of pre and post natal services and in all aspects of health education.

Dear old G.M. Smith had acknowledged the important role they played in his overall plan and treated his nurses as though they were house surgeons at-large. His nurses had no need to prescribe medicines - he saw to it that they were well stocked with the basic drugs needed in their situation. This practice of giving nurses such autonomy met with considerable criticism from his old enemy - the Health Department. Yet nobody came up with a better plan, given the geography of the region. Some nurses found the expectation to practice their profession according to the circumstances they confronted involved a level of professional responsibility that they could not accept and they soon resigned. Others thrived on this freedom and served in the district for the greater part of their working lives. Their constant presence, by living among them, was deeply appreciated by the communities they served and *their* nurse enjoyed a level of respect equalled by few other residents. Many nurses married into the district and still continued their professional lives, thus breaking with the tedious tradition that marriage dictated an end to a nursing career.

Most New Zealand nursing graduates at first found conditions in the Hokianga something of a culture shock, whereas those from overseas were often totally overwhelmed by the experience. New appointees usually began work either in the hospital, or within the Rawene district, so that they would have both support and supervision for the first few weeks.

I had been at Rawene a couple of weeks when a nurse from Britain arrived on the railway bus to take up a position with us. She was a petite, sparkling young lady who would not have been out of place at a Government House reception.

Renee attended to her welcome, initiation and grand tour. I was surprised at the Matron's enthusiasm for a new staff member who appeared to be so clearly out of her depth in the earthy basics of the Hokianga. Surely, with all her experience, Renee could read the signs.

Proof of the pudding came the next day when a request for a visit was made from a remote household while I was attending a clinic on the other side of the harbour. Our fashion-page model, now sartorially subdued by her nurse's uniform, was despatched with the hospital car, her bag of supplies and a map, with instructions to proceed to the end of a certain road where she would find transport waiting to carry her the mile or so to the house.

A closed farm gate separated the deteriorating public road from a deeply rutted, narrow tractor-track that lead to the house nestling in the valley. She parked the car and awaited the guttural chug-chug of a tractor that she anticipated would carry her the rest of the way.

After half an hour of silence she decided to stretch her legs. The only other living thing around was a horse grazing casually near the gate. The animal bore a sack on its back with something white attached to this basic cover. She decided to check out the animal and wandered over. The white patch turned out to be a scrap of note paper attached by a safety pin. On the paper was written, "For the nurse."

She promptly gathered up her bag, moved the horse alongside the gate and used the latter to mount the animal. Obediently the horse turned down the track and carried |her gently to the homestead. That nurse stayed on for years serving the Hokianga with distinction.

This capacity to readily adapt to the circumstances in which they find themselves was the hallmark of all the nurses and doctors who served the Hokianga Special Area.

I was reminded of this many years later when I encounted a photograph of Renee in the glossy social pages of the old 'Weekly News'. After her retirement she had been awarded, in the Honours List, appropriate recognition of her outstanding services to nursing. There she stood at the Vice-Regal Reception, proudly gazing out from the page, complete with picture-hat and gloves. Renee had responded confidently to the social challenge and did so with dignity and taste. No doubt she was impatient to get home and shed the trappings of convention, but for the meantime she was prepared to conform. This she owed to herself, her profession and those who had served with her. I loved her for it.

I was in my third month at Rawene when word came through that relief was at hand. It arrived in the form of Bernie Bowden. Bernie was ready to go to the UK to complete his studies in Ophthalmology and while waiting for his passage was seeking employment. (Eventually he would return to Whangarei as our Ophthalmologist.)

He arrived while I was away attending clinics, so I met him in the staff room in the evening. It was the usual scene. The Priest was there together with a handful of off duty nurses and a smattering of relatives supporting sick family members. We had hardly settled down to chat when Renee, with eyes a flutter, burst into the room to announce that a local farmer had a cow with a deeply lacerated leg that needed urgent attention. Bernie responded with characteristic enthusiasm and Renee was delighted. I knew then that the new man would be OK and confidently left the room to pack my bags.

The journey back to the relative civilisation of Whangarei was uneventful. However, I noted with some concern that passing Whangarei motorists consistently failed to respond to my casual wave. It took a couple of weeks for me to omit the gestures of acknowledgement that had become a Hokianga habit.

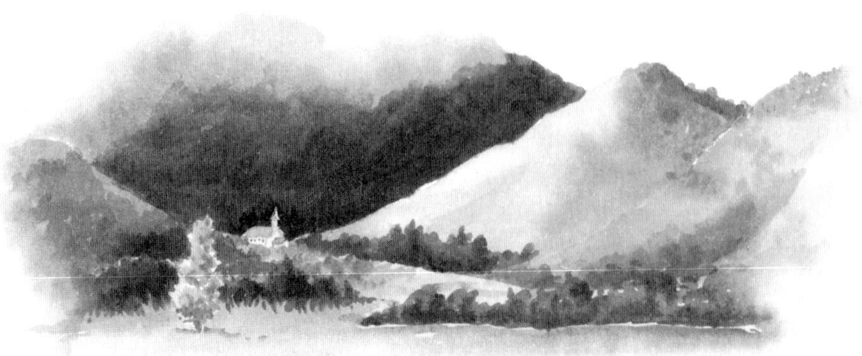

Church South Hokianga.

HANDS ACROSS THE SEA

I was glad to be back because I had a small yacht moored in the Town Basin, which I was working on in my spare time and this project had been neglected during my absence.

Wednesday afternoon was my afternoon off and I was busy at the moorings when a local G.P. and hospital anaesthetist, Lou Simmonds, called in to observe my workmanship. (I had learned long before that if you want free advice try planting a garden or work on a boat.)

Lou, who was also Port Health Officer, informed me that he was standing-by to take part in a rescue mission. A lighthouse keeper on Moko Hinau Island - miles off the coast from Whangarei - had possibly suffered a heart attack and was due to be picked up from the island that afternoon by the British destroyer Concord. Lou was to go out on the Harbour Board launch Oleo to meet the destroyer beyond the three mile limit and take off the patient. Would I like to come? He assured me there was plenty of room on the launch and if I had any friends who would like a trip, we should meet at the wharf before four-thirty.

I assured him of my determination to join in and continued with the renovations. Before long Dr. Pullar, the local eye specialist, turned up to offer supervision and advice. Yes he would love to come and promised to be down at the wharf on time.

As the afternoon wore on the prospect of adventure on the high sea warmed with the weather and I began to think of others who might enjoy this unique outing. My friend Jo came to mind. She had a flat nearby, was a teacher and should be home from school in time to participate. Her response was both positive and immediate, but in the excitement she managed to twist her ankle, eventually joining the ship's company with a painful limp.

By four-thirty M.V. Oleo, a solidly built, workhorse of a boat, was alive with activity. Her two man crew had the engine idling in anticipation as the motley assortment of hangers-on settled in and patiently waited for the show to begin.

The vessel's ship-to-shore radio crackled with static as we maintained a listening watch, plotting the progress of Concord as she steamed at full power from Tauranga having broken off from manoeuvres to engage in this mission of mercy.

Suddenly lines were cast, the gentle diesel throb accelerated through to a powerful growl and we were under way to meet a British destroyer on the high seas.

The sun was low when we cleared the heads and lay to anchor in Smugglers Cove awaiting further contact with Concord. Oleo rose and fell on a gentle ocean swell as we gathered around the crackling radio with ears tuned for further developments.

When the voice came it was very loud, clear and distinctly British.

"Concord to Oleo - Concord to Oleo - are you receiving - over."

The cold, clipped, precision of the man froze Oleo's complement for a moment and then galvanised our radio operator into inspired action.

"Er - yes - ah - Oleo to Concord - er - got ya - er - over."

The crisp accent returned immediately carrying with it the awe and authority of the entire British Navy.

"Concord to Oleo - Concord to Oleo - have you doctor on board - over."

Our man nervously scanned the assembled company and with a hint of panic replied -

"Er - Oleo to Concord - ah - we have three doctors on board - er - over."

The British Navy was clearly impressed with the magnitude of the medical response in this endeavour and there was a long pause while the significance of the message percolated through the destroyer's hierarchy.

"Concord to Oleo - Concord to Oleo - please repeat - please repeat - over."

To have the credibility of his communiqué questioned in this way both annoyed and flustered our man, who had come to resent the presence of his joy riding audience. He grabbed the microphone and shouted -

"Three bloody doctors."

Concord's reply was prompt and tinged with a little respect - after all, Oleo almost certainly had more doctors on board than they had.

"Concord to Oleo - Concord to Oleo - message understood - three er doctors - over." And the radio fell back into a crackle-studded silence.

I went on deck to adjust the fluid balance between myself and the Pacific Ocean. Darkness was gathering and a single unblinking light shone from far out to sea. Within a minute it was three lights that quickly grew into a dozen. Concord was dashing towards us. I called the others and we watched the ship grow into a block of well illuminated, multi-storeyed buildings in the time it took to raise Oleo's anchor. She stood patiently just outside the three mile limit while we chugged over to join her.

As we slid across the black sea, drawn towards the glittering spectacle of a destroyer standing stock still, the business of taking off a patient seemed to be a simple matter, but as we came alongside this colossus the first problem became obvious. The long, low six foot swell that bore Oleo made no impression on the warship. She simply stood there as though rooted to the sea floor while we regularly rose and fell through a couple of metres.

The second problem involved Oleo. There was no clear space on her cabin top to land a stretcher. Her wheelhouse, exhaust funnel, mast and towing bollard all broke up the upper surface of the vessel. Furthermore her cabin entrance was very close to and overlooked the stern.

Concord's entire crew lined every handrail and filled every porthole to watch the procedure as powerful spotlights illuminated the scene below. We were contemplating our problems in silence when a British sailor, distracted momentarily by a small crisis of his own, was moved to exclaim - "Buggar!"

Immediately a fellow mariner, dismayed by this sudden indiscretion, loudly reprimanded its author -

"Shut your bloody mouth, can't you see there is a bloody woman down there."

Worse things can happen at sea.

With our patient strapped into a stretcher and dangling from several decks above, we prepared to catch him in that moment when Oleo was arrested in the trough of the swell and before she rose once more - then slip him head first through the cabin entrance and onto the cabin floor in one unbroken movement. At that moment Concord's crew had to slack off the suspending ropes before he was either dropped into the sea or jerked away from us. (At this stage it occurred to me that if he hadn't already suffered a heart attack, he could well have one any minute.)

With all hands in position the manoeuvre went like clockwork and the terrified patient lay safely on the cabin floor as we backed away and turned for home aglow with self satisfaction. Oleo's crew, who had previously been a little irritated by us sightseers, were by now grateful for the extra hands that the venture had attracted (and were gracious enough to say so.) In the time it took to cover the three miles to the harbour entrance, Concord had disappeared over the horizon.

Fortunately, it turned out that our patient was not as ill as had been feared - indeed it is possible that Jo, with her sprained ankle, was probably the most serious case involved in the entire exercise.

ONCE BITTEN

Sometimes the sea contributes to human accidents in strange ways. There was the case of a lady who had most of the tendons on the top of her foot lacerated by a stingray. Fred took great interest in this case and used it to teach us the finer points of tendon repair.

And then there was the incident in which a fisherman was bitten by a shark. He arrived at outpatients in a very agitated state with a series of parallel lacerations on either side of his thigh. Despite the history, the wounds were surprisingly superficial and easily repaired. As the suturing proceeded he explained the circumstances with some embarrassment.

He was fishing alone when he hooked a sizeable shark and decided to bring the catch home (shark liver enjoyed a good market in those days). With some difficulty he managed to stun the brute and eventually had his catch draped across the poop deck and lashed there in the best tradition of deepsea fishing launches. During the journey back up the harbour, while standing in the cockpit he stepped back, placing his thigh inside the open jaws of his trussed up trophy. The fish had just enough residual energy to gently close its jaws as its victim pulled away in terror.

In due course the notes on the case were filed under 'accidental injury', 'cause of injury - shark bite'. Many years later someone compiled a chronological review of shark attack in New Zealand's waters, listing Whangarei Harbour as on of the many danger spots the author identified around our shores. The date of the event enabled me to identify this particular incident as the one I had dealt with. One could hardly equate putting ones leg into the open mouth of a half dead shark as shark attack - which raises the question of just how useful (or dangerous) such poorly researched data really is.

KAITAIA

FRIENDLY NATIVES

The second year at Whangarei was drawing to a close, when I heard that Kaitaia Hospital (a good one hundred miles north of Whangarei) had a new Superintendent - one Bob Spencer. Bob and his wife Barbara had spent a couple of years in China with Rewi Alley establishing a hospital in the Gobi Desert before he went to England to complete his post graduate studies in General Surgery. The good news was that he was looking for an assistant and would I like the job? I took it.

Moving to Kaitaia would have been a straight forward business if it had not included the boat. Christmas holidays were earmarked for the voyage and the only chart of the coastline from Whangarei to North Cape was purchased and studied. The survey on which the chart was based was made in the late nineteenth century. It showed Kaitaia as 'Kaitaia Mission Station' and offered the comforting observation - 'Friendly Natives'.

The voyage was probably the most poorly planned maritime adventure of the decade - punctuated as it was by extremes of weather and gross miscalculations. The fact that it was eventually completed had more to do with the benevolence of Divine Providence than seamanship. I was finally emboldened to undertake the venture when a friend, who had considerable coastal sailing experience and a few days to spare at the right time, offered to join Jo and I in the trip.

We set out in glorious sunshine and little wind. Despite the pleasant weather there was a steep ocean swell - the sort that often precedes a north-easterly storm. By early afternoon we had crept well up the coast with every prospect of clearing Cape Brett comfortably before sunset, when the horizon beyond the Cape began to darken ominously and our favourable breeze died away in grim anticipation. Further progress north was now out of the question. It was time to reef down and prepare to dash for shelter. The north-easterly came in on cue, filling the sails and driving us along in a flurry of foam and spray towards Tutukaka and shelter. We shot through the narrow harbour entrance as angry seas smashed in frustration against the cliffs and the first of the rain peppered down.

A blackened sky swallowed up the daylight as a monsoon of rain hammered wildly on the decks and set the sea a-tremble. Spontaneous, muddy waterfalls cascaded down the surrounding hillsides and drummed into the bay all night while a frustrated wind howled in the rigging.

Next morning, folk on a deep-sea fishing launch moored close by, informed us that if we wanted to go to Kaitaia we would need a boat because all the roads to the town were now closed by slips or flooding and its main street was under several feet of water.

The storm raged on, eating away the time our friend and mentor had laid aside for the journey. Expressing deep regret he had to return home, leaving Jo and I to make the next decision.

On the third day the storm eased and the sea relaxed. With favourable winds restored, we decided to make a run for it and set off in the late afternoon to retrace our steps to Cape Brett. Guided by the Brett light we crept on through the night and by sunset next day we were riding to anchor in Deep Water Cove and dined on snapper caught with our last rasher of bacon.

The following day dawned oily calm. We wallowed, slack-sailed, until late morning before the wind filled in from the south-west and carried us up the coast at a pleasing clip. At sunset we entered what I had predicted to be Doubtless Bay, except that off to the east was a large island. Could I be mistaken? Was this really part of the Cavalli Islands that I thought had passed well to seaward hours ago? Yet there it was - one big island that had to be accounted for. In the gathering darkness and with the promise of a moon soon to rise, we sailed on.

A gentle off-shore breeze edged us along through the night creeping between the mainland and the mystery island. After a couple of hours of pleasant sailing, a new sound intruded above the gurgling of our wake - the rumble of surf on a not too distant shore. At the same time the boat began to slowly rise and fall confirming our proximity to a beach. Gybing immediately we retraced our path to safer waters and prudently anchored for the remainder of the night.

Dawn restored our island just where we had left it and in the early morning haze we set out to repeat the night's journey. As we slipped along, a sandspit slowly grew out from the island and another emerged from the mainland. Within an hour the morning mist had cleared and the sandspits joined up to become a continuous shore.

We had been in Doubtless Bay all along and our island was really Cape Karekare linked to the mainland by a long, low, sandy peninsular which simply became lost in the haze at sunrise and sunset.

I had hoped to get the boat to Awanui on the Rangunu Harbour, but this plan had to be abandoned when we attempted to sail around Cape Karekare. A wind shift threatened us with a dangerous lee shore, so we returned to Doubtless Bay and finally anchored in Mangonui Harbour. This journey probably made us the last settlers in the district to arrive by sailing ship.

ASK JIM TAAFFE

For the meantime I was able to borrow a mooring at Mill Bay while I cast about to set up my own. To do this I needed a length of chain - a commodity in short supply in the late fifties. The first person I asked for guidance in this matter thought for a while and then suggested -

"Ask Jim Taaffe."

This did not seem to be very helpful so I made the rounds of hardware shops and at each the story was the same.

"Sorry mate, chain's hard to get these days - have you tried Jim Taaffe?"

So I tried Jim Taaffe. I rang him, introduced myself and explained my problem. He confirmed what I had already learned about the current availability of chain and then helpfully suggested I leave it to him.

A day or so later he rang back to say he had found some chain and knew of someone who would put a mooring down for me. And that's the way it was in Kaitaia - if you had a problem you couldn't solve you asked Jim Taaffe.

Onetime chairman of the local Town Board and later first Mayor of Kaitaia, Jim had established a transport empire in Kaitaia after returning from the First World War. He ran busses, trucks and taxis and also retailed petrol. Jim regularly combed Ninety Mile Beach like a magpie and had sheds full of the flotsam and jetsam he had gathered over the years.

Jim was a Justice of the Peace, District Coroner and Marriage Conciliator. You could say he was Kaitaia's number one citizen and his address was unique:-

"J.T.B. TAAFFE J.P.
No. 1 Taaffe St.
Phone 1
Box 1
Kaitaia

He was also the official certifying officer for ambergris. This peculiar, grey, waxy material is believed to begin life as the beak of a giant squid, which has been partially digested in the stomach of a sperm whale. The whale eventually releases the ambergris leaving it free to float ashore.

The perfume industry use it to retain fragrances in their products. It used to be auctioned in Paris once each year, thus establishing its market value for the next twelve months. Even in the late fifties, finders could deposit ambergris in trading banks - its value determined by the previous Paris auction price.

Before a piece of ambergris could be credited to an account, the bank would weigh the material and record the result. A copy of this weight would be given to the prospective depositor, who would then be directed to a certifier who would re-weigh the piece to confirm its identity and issue a certificate recording the test results.

Testing consisted of heating an iron nail in a candle flame and then plunging the hot metal into the substance in question. The characteristic sweet, musty odour released by this process would confirm its true nature.

Jim shared number one Taaffe Street with his wife, affectionately know as 'Sweet.' She had the uncanny ability to be able to smell ambergris at a distance. I recall being at their home when a visitor called. She answered his knock and advised the stranger on the doorstep that Jim was out at the moment but it was indeed ambergris he was carrying and Jim would confirm this for him if he returned later in the afternoon.

Being number one citizen, Jim was keen to be the first in the district to own any new appliance - and so it was with washing machines. They had the first electric washing machine in town - an agitator model - with a power driven wringer that could be swung over the bowl.

Their daughter was doing some washing with the new acquisition when home alone. The scarf she was wearing became caught up in the wringer, choking her to death.

This shattering tragedy was made even worse for Jim and Sweet by the cold, legal formality of the Coroner's Court, where the subsequent hearing into the death was held. He determined then, that should he ever become Coroner, families caught up in tragic deaths would have their cases heard in the unthreatening and humane atmosphere of a normal sitting room.

I attended several Coroner's hearings at number one Taaffe Street, presided over by Jim, seated around the dining table with police in attendance (armed with the family bible for the necessary swearing) while witnesses and the family involved were seated in arm chairs. Sweet would be out in the kitchen, buttering fresh scones to be served with tea when the proceedings were concluded. It was a gentle business that could not, for practical reasons, be sustained by subsequent incumbents, but at least some families benefited from this sensitive, unorthodox, innovation in legal procedure.

Being a Coroner in a community with a large Maori population made Jim very sensitive to Maori expectations and he did everything in his power to achieve the early release of bodies that fell within his jurisdiction. His reputation in this matter was deeply appreciated by the Maori community and in this regard J.T.B. Taaffe J.P. was half a century ahead of his fellow Coroners, who are only now acknowledging the importance of this aspect of cultural sensitivity. Those of us who performed post mortem examinations under his orders were always urged to proceed as soon as possible, while he stood by to enable the tangi to proceed immediately the findings were at hand.

KAITAIA

Long before Europeans invaded this country, Kaitaia (although under a different name) supported a stable Maori community. An influential chief in the district during the early days of colonisation was Nopera Panakareao. Impressed with Christianity and realising that European contact brought with it European goods, he was anxious to see the Church Missionary Society (Church of England) extend its activities into his territory. To this end he made several journeys to the Bay of Islands and eventually convinced a party of missionaries (that included William Puckey and Joseph Matthews) to make a tour of the Far North in 1832.

They visited many places between Whangaroa and Ninety Mile Beach but Panakareao had a deal for them that they could not resist. He had timber laid aside for buildings and appropriate land (about a thousand acres) earmarked for purchase. With this tempting package came his guarantee of protection. In this way he won the day and two years later land was purchased and the mission station established. It was Puckey and Matthews who chose the name 'Kaitaia' and the two families settled down to their long and difficult task.

My old chart was correct "Kaitaia Mission Station - friendly natives." Governor Hobson dropped in while gathering autographs on his 1840 Treaty of Waitangi and collected sixty in Kaitaia covering both Te Rarawa and Te Aupouri tribes. It was at this gathering that Nopera Panakareao carried the day with his oft quoted observation that only 'the shadow of the land is to the Queen, but the substance remains to us.' An opinion that he would reverse within a year.

The chief remained a dedicated supporter of the Anglican Mission and is buried, not in his tribal burial grounds, but in a distant corner of the church graveyard - at the alter site of the first church - a decision that must have been difficult for some of his family and followers to accept.

Kauri gum and dairy farming drew European settlers north to begin new lives in the shadow of the Kaitaia Mission. The commerce, that followed in the wake of such settlement, became established in an old river flat below the Mission Station. The various offices, banks and stores stretched out along an ancient pathway like willows on the bank of a stream. This central roadway was appropriately named Commerce Street. On either side and parallel with Commerce Street the pioneering missionary families of Puckey and Matthews are commemorated in street names. Nopea Panakareao's name lives on as a short, blind street that extends across the front of the Anglican Church.

Kaitaia remained a rather remote, inland community for about a hundred years after the mission was established - until a passable road through the Mangamuka Gorge linked the embryonic town with the rest of the country. The 'boom years' followed. This late developer was soon challenging the nearby port of Mangonui and by 1934 the Mangonui Hospital (est. 1907) had been dismantled and reassembled in Kaitaia. Nopea Panakareao put 'Kaitaia' on the map - Puckey and Matthews kept it there.

A LANKY TEENAGER

At first glance Kaitaia Hospital reminded me of a lanky teenager who was rapidly outgrowing his clothes. Originally the kauri main building stood overlooking the harbour at Mangonui some twenty odd miles away. Because the population of that district was falling steadily in the thirties and briskly growing in Kaitaia and Awanui, the decision was taken to cut the Mangonui building into sections, load it onto barges and ship it across Doubtless Bay, around Cape Karekare and thence via Awanui to Kaitaia where it was reassembled on a hill safely above the morning mist and overlooking the town.

By mid century the hospital was once again too small to satisfy the needs of the local population and improvisation was called for - something that my new boss, Bob Spencer, was very good at.

Now, as part of New Zealand's defence preparations during the Second World War, thousands of 'army huts' were built to house our soldiers and their equipment in preparation for the much feared Japanese invasion that did not come for another thirty years and when it did it was so subtle that few recognised it.

After the war these huts were sold off and for a couple of decades became ubiquitous building units dedicated either to housing or storage, according to need.

Army huts were built to one plan - eight feet by twelve (that's nearly four metres by almost three). By knocking out the appropriate sides or ends, they could be combined, like so many building blocks, to form large and complex structures.

Bob, inspired by their inherent adaptability, arranged for a series of these huts to be linked together to create a barely adequate ward for children - thus relieving some of the pressure on the adult accommodation. Each carpenter involved in the exercise must have worked independently resulting in an overall floor that undulated alarmingly - and a complex roofing system that leaked regularly.

The much adapted main building struggled to contain the new services required of it - despite the space liberated when the children were moved out. The X-ray Department occupied what was formerly a two-bed sideroom and boasted an ancient machine donated to the hospital many years previously by the Archibald family. The newly established laboratory began in a large storage cupboard that opened onto the main corridor. (Fortunately the fist incumbent, Ron McKenzie, was of modest stature.) By cutting the cupboard door into two, horizontally, the top half could be opened for ventilation and the bottom section provided access for the lone technician.

Bob Spencer was the prime cause of this sudden expansion and congestion. After a long history of medical officers on short term or temporary appointments, the community suddenly found itself with an enthusiastic and competent surgeon. Word soon spread around the saleyards and across the bowling greens that the new man was an energetic young surgeon who thrived on work and enjoyed a laugh with anyone.

Giant hernias, that had barely been contained by sweaty, tatty, trusses and had been concealed in trousers with some difficulty for years, suddenly saw the light of day. Gall stones that had grumbled and groaned for decades had now found a hand that could be trusted to remove them.

The new-found confidence in the hospital spread like measles through a boarding school and filled the Outpatient Clinics. Previously hidden pathology was smuggled into waiting rooms and the operating lists grew steadily longer.

Despite this surge in demand we never had a waiting list that was not determined by the individual. Dairy farmers arranged for their operations to be done during the 'dry season' - commercial fishers when their boat was due for survey - commercial travellers from Auckland booked in according to their annual leave and kids were dealt with during school holidays. The whole system revolved around a modest pocket diary (courtesy of the May and Baker drug company) that lived in Bob's long white coat pocket.

Apart from the wooden main building and the Third World children's ward, the hospital grounds also contained a stand-alone wooden maternity unit, a nurses home, an isolated T.B. shelter and sundry buildings dedicated as outpatient clinics. A boiler house, laundry and kitchen completed the establishment.

When I arrived, the hospital gardens were still functioning - but only just. A small valley just beyond the boiler house had been cultivated for decades to supply fresh vegetables and at one stage, laying hens were kept on site as well as a milking cow, replaced regularly by a sympathetic farmer. Escalating labour costs and diminishing soil fertility contrived to bring to an end this quaint, though healthy, tradition.

Although in the mid thirties the first Labour Government had taken over the financing of hospitals, the community at large still considered their hospital to be a worthy charity when it came to the disposal of excess food. This was a hangover from the days when hospitals were maintained through local body rates and any reduction in their running costs could be reflected in an easing of rate demands. The catch from a particularly successful fishing trip was commonly shared in this way. This would remain so until the domestic freezer became a common household item.

I well remember a very busy night on duty that was finally under control by the early morning. As I wearily trudged down the darkened corridor anticipating a little sleep, I encountered a lone figure heading towards me. My heart sank at the prospect of more traumatised citizens - and rose again when I discovered that the greatest problem on the horizon was the need to get three giant Hapuka (Grouper) from the back of his truck and into the hospital kitchen cool store.

Food, then as now, was also a common raffle prize. A couple of weeks after I began work at Kaitaia Hospital I was approached by a nurse to buy a raffle ticket in support of her basketball club. To prove what a good sport she was dealing with, I had parted with the cash and accepted the appropriate documentation before I had even asked about the potential prize.

"First prize is six frozen native pigeons - the second is four - third is two."

In my youth I had been a junior member of 'Forest and Bird' and was now praying that I would not be disgraced by holding a winning ticket.

THE MILK OF PARADISE

Bob, although familiar with the primitive conditions that prevailed in the Gobi Desert of China, was appalled, on arrival in Kaitaia, to find that the hospital kitchen was serving raw milk to the patients. Pasteurised milk had not reached the town, and country folk, especially the kids, had no stomach for the taste of scalded milk.

His first task was to find someone who could construct a small pasteurisation plant for the hospital kitchen. That someone was the hospital engineer Bonnar Wright - the quintessential Kiwi innovator. He promptly created and installed a make-shift pasteurisation plant that would have done credit to Heath Robinson.

The local newspaper ran the story of the hospital's latest acquisition, but the article failed to inspire the authorities to review their position on the pasteurisation of the town milk supply. Instead they published further recommendations that emphasised the wisdom of boiling milk for human consumption - and the kids continued to avoid drinking it. What was needed at this stage was proof that the town's raw milk supply was indeed a public health hazard.

Bob engaged Adrian Webb, our T.B. specialist, in the problem when he next visited from Whangarei and together they developed a strategy. Each month Adrian held an outpatient's clinic for children with T.B. glands in their necks. Here the infection was believed to enter via the tonsils and was presumed to indicate that T.B. contaminated milk had been ingested. (Indeed at one time it was common practice to send all tonsils removed at tonsillectomy to the pathologist to exclude active T.B. infection). Certainly there were plenty of kids attending his clinic, but because they moved freely between town and country it was not possible to determine whether the infection arose from the town supply or from milk encountered on a relative's farm. Farm milk had always been viewed with more suspicion than the milk delivered to the town.

Adrian then embarked on a survey of T.B. reactors among the pupils of Kaitaia College. This would indicate the number of students who, at some stage in their lives, had been in contact with T.B. from whatever source. Most of the reactors would have overcome the initial infection by natural healing and follow up chest x-rays would exclude current active disease.

At first glance the results were not very informative. The incidence of positive reactors was only a little above the national average, so it had to be presumed that the milk supply could not be incriminated on these figures alone.

Most health professionals were convinced that Kaitaia's milk supply was highly suspect, but proof was still lacking. At this stage Adrian had a bright idea and returned to his list of college reactors and separated them into two groups - those who lived within the boundaries of the town and were thus exposed to the town milk supply every day and those who lived out in the countryside and almost exclusively drank farm milk. Although the college roll was divided equally between town and country, nearly every reactor had a town address. Thus the farmer's house cow was producing vastly safer milk than the town supply - a result that very few had predicted. The reason was simple. Farmers selected their healthiest animal as 'house cow' but the town milk was pooled from several farms and hundreds of cows.

At last the case was proven and under the weight of this evidence, plus some direct pressure from the Health Department, the authorities reluctantly agreed to introduce pasteurisation.

Before the victory could be celebrated, the Dairy Workers Union stepped in, demanding a staffing level for the proposed plant that the town fathers insisted would be financially crippling.

Things were at this stage when I arrived and stood at my gate with my billy, waiting for the milkman with his can and dipper, to call and bail out a couple of pints of the raw stuff. The pasteurisation plant was now trapped between the union's manning expectations and the employers reluctance to meet the proposed wage bill - and there it stayed, unresolved.

Late one afternoon I had a call from a local G.P. He wished to admit a child of about three and a half who was proving to be a significant behaviour problem. The child's parents - he explained apologetically - were going through some pretty intense relationship problems in Auckland and the patient had been brought north, a few weeks earlier, to stay with relatives during the parental crisis. He added that over the past few days the youngster's behaviour had steadily deteriorated - alternating between determined aggression when disturbed and profound withdrawal when left alone. This paradoxical pattern of behaviour was driving the caring relatives to distraction. They, and the G.P., attributed this reaction to a psychological response arising from the tension between the parents. The expectation was that once the child had settled down in hospital all would come right - which seemed to me to be a very long shot.

The child was admitted. I soon discovered that it was impossible to make a physical examination without stimulating very determined resistance, but the moment everyone withdrew the child curled up and lay quite still. The attempt to examine the child was an obvious failure. So far, all I had to go on was a clinical picture that could be summed up as 'angry-lethargy'. This was the old fashioned name given by the physicians of yesteryear to Infantile Tuberculous Meningitis.

Ron confirmed the diagnosis from his broom-cupboard laboratory and I sat down with the distraught relatives to break the bad news and try to work out where the T.B. had come from. There was no family history of the disease and at the age of three and a half the infant had little chance to make significant contact with T.B. infected strangers. However, during the few weeks it had lived in Kaitaia the infant had been drinking raw milk. Furthermore the infant's uncle worked at the town supply plant where workers and management remained deadlocked over the newly installed pasteurisation plant.

Within days the dispute was resolved and the first bottles of pasteurised milk hit the streets of Kaitaia. Three months later the clinic for children with T.B. glands of the neck was closed when the supply of patients dried up. Bonnar Wright carefully dismantled his pride and joy in the hospital kitchen and thoughtfully squirreled away the bits and pieces - you never know when they might come in handy.

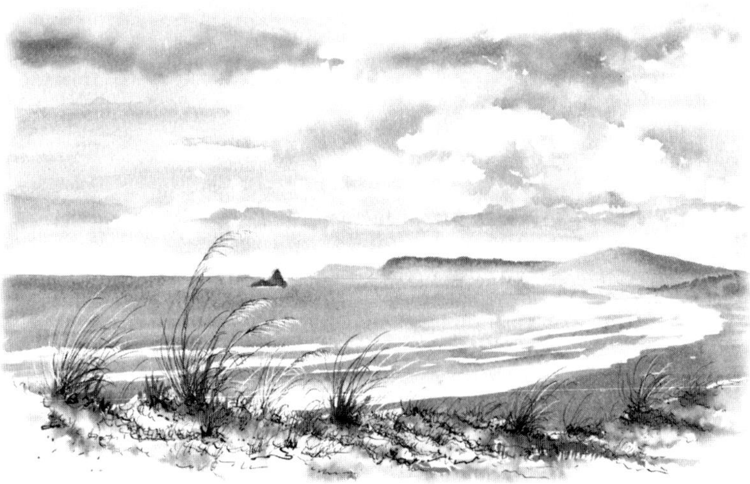

Ninety Mile Beach from the Bluff.

LAUDABLE PUS

Today's friendly family surgeon came to us courtesy of the local barber. In 1506 the Barber-Surgeons of Edinburgh received their royal charter from James IV of Scotland. Forty years later Henry VIII of England similarly recognised the Barber-Surgeons Company of London which, in time, evolved into the Royal College of Surgeons. The thing about barbers was they were very good at sharpening things - a skill greatly appreciated by the general public.

The barber's pole, with its double spiral of red and white bears mute testimony to the blood and bandages associated with their calling. The perverse insistence of today's surgeon on being addressed as plain old Mr., Mrs. or Miss is really a distant echo of their ancient craft-guild origins. Although surgeons may be called upon to carve the meat for a dinner party, they are never approached for a haircut.

Surgery in Central Europe had different origins. After Andreas Vesalius had published his remarkable text on human anatomy in Padua in 1543, Central European surgeons found an academic basis for their profession that owed nothing to barbers. The protracted wars that followed the Reformation flooded Europe with wounded soldiers and offered surgeons abundant opportunities to dress wounds, amputate limbs and write textbooks.

One such surgeon-author was Ambrose Pare who made a great study of his profession in France and is credited with establishing the foundation of modern surgery. Pare was an observant man. He noted that if pus formed in a wound there was a good chance the patient would survive and eventually heal. This observation of hope lead him to coin the phrase 'laudable pus'. Seen in the light of today's expectations for wound healing, the phrase 'laudable pus' becomes an oxymoron.

Despite the implied contradiction, these pioneer surgeons had a point. Wound healing depends on an adequate blood supply and in situations where that supply is compromised, the tissue is quickly invaded by the organisms that create 'gas gangrene' and the fatal toxins associated with it. In these circumstances pus is not created and death is swift, silent and peaceful.

A good blood supply, on the other hand, inhibits the gangrene bugs through a raised oxygen level and supplies the plasma and white blood cells that contribute the bulk of the laudable fluid. Although they had got it wrong, they had done so for the right reasons.

A number of different bacteria can stimulate the production of pus, but one of the commonest contaminants rejoices under the imposing title of Staphylococcus aureus - so named because under the microscope it resembles small, round, berry-like structures (that's the 'coccus' bit) gathered in clumps resembling miniature bunches of grapes (that's the 'staph' bit). Aureus, a golden Roman coin once worth twenty five denarii, refers to the golden colour of the colonies when the bacterium is cultured in the laboratory. This is the bug most commonly involved in boils, abscesses and most wound infections. We all carry it around on our skin and up our noses with careless abandon.

Problems begin for us when it gets *under* our skin, either through trauma or surgery - or via the ducts of skin glands (giving boils) or into the biggest modified sweat glands of all - mammary tissue, giving breast abscesses. If enough staphylococci get into the blood stream it can create abscesses (pockets of pus) almost anywhere.

Staph. aureus has probably been in Europe for centuries, but did it occur in the Pacific before European exploration and subsequent invasion? Diseases from Europe, in the end, caused more carnage among colonised indigenous people than European weapons ever did. T.B., smallpox, measles, influenza, typhoid, gonorrhoea and syphilis all took their tragic toll. The question is - did Staphylococcus areus come with them?

When Captain Cook explored the Pacific on his first voyage, he witnessed the New Zealand Maori ceremony of tattooing and described the experience in his journal. However, on his second visit his request to once again observe the Maori practice of this art was firmly declined. Legend suggests that since contact with Europeans the Maori were dismayed to find that many tattoos went 'bad'. This experience could suggest that a new factor had been introduced and this intruder could well be the Staphylococcus organism. Today, of course, we claim to be one people with the staph. bug on everyone's skin and up all noses.

Should the ubiquitous staph. find its way into the blood stream of a reasonably healthy person, the patient's white cells would usually clean it up as long as they gained good access to the offending organism. However, some situations exist where the bug may settle in and gain the upper hand. One such locus is found inside the growing ends of adolescent bones. Here the bone ends enjoy a very rich blood supply made up of narrow blood vessels tangled together like a bundle of miniature spaghetti. These vessels are narrow enough to entrap a cluster of Staph. aureus - precipitating a fierce local battle. Technically we now have an expanding boil trapped within a rigid casing of bone. The condition is known as acute osteomyelitis. Here pain is intense, fever is high and the patient quickly becomes gravely ill.

Staph. aureus is a bit like gorse. Apart from their shared golden flowering, both exhibit modest growth when in cooler climates, but in sub-tropical latitudes their growth is prone to accelerate beyond control. Thus, in Dunedin, osteomyelitis is an uncommon condition, yet in Whangarei we would admit a new case every two or three months, despite the much smaller population.

During one weekend in Kaitaia I admitted two adolescent lads with osteomyelitis of the upper end of the femur. In those days the patient would be in theatre under a general anaesthetic within an hour or so of admission and antibiotics would be withheld until a sample of the pus had been taken for culture.

Once the offending bone end had been exposed, a series of holes were drilled into the bone using a sterilised version of a carpenter's hand drill with a bit about as thick as the legendary number eight fencing wire. A swab would be taken from the pus that surged up through the first drill hole. The drilling would be repeated at one centimetre intervals down the bone, stopping when the last two holes released blood instead of pus. In effect a bone abscess was being drained.

When penicillin was first used, staphylococci were very sensitive to it and the pioneer antibiotic was hailed as a 'miracle drug'. However, within a few years this organism was developing resistance to penicillin and tarnishing the miracle.

The race was now on to find new antibiotics faster than this bacterium could develop resistance to those already in use. By the early sixties the golden Staphylococcus was ahead of the pharmaceutical companies and the new, totally resistant strain, was dubbed the 'H bug'. The 'H' referring to 'hospital' - the environment in which this 'killer' strain had developed. (Eventually new antibiotics overcame this dangerous impasse and the 'H bug' threat evaporated until in recent years Staphylococcus aureus once again achieved total resistance. The new variant is dignified by the more upmarket acronym 'M.R.S.A'.)

In Kaitaia, in the sixties, an alarming number of cases of osteomyelitis yielded bugs that were resistant to most of the current antibiotics, yet the patients involved had had little direct contact with hospitals. However, many of them came from farms where antibiotics were common place in every milking shed. In a district where prosperity depended on the twice daily emptying of a cow's udder, episodes of mastitis significantly eroded farm profit and farmers were prepared to pay good money for the latest antibiotics in order to keep ahead.

Other people's 'H bug' was our 'farm bug' and we could see the day approaching when totally antibiotic resistant staphylococci could be created in the milking shed and spread from there to the farmer and his family.

Fortunately, in our community, it was easy to control the situation because the whole district was served by only two vets and they alone prescribed all farm antibiotic remedies. Both readily agreed to withhold one major antibiotic from veterinary use until new antibiotics entered the market.

In the early sixties Bob and I spent a lot of time releasing 'laudable pus' from abscesses. The most common sites were the groins of children (following infection of sores on the legs that had ascended along the lymphatic system) and the breasts of lactating women. Indeed a visiting colleague, after surveying our cases, wrote us off as the 'suppurating North' and maybe he had a point.

As the seventies rolled on the incidence of staphylococcal infection eased. Maybe the bug had simply lost some of its virulence or perhaps, as the modern bathroom-shower succeeded over the weekly soak in a tub, our personal population of golden staph. took a beating.

BURNT SKIN

For a district that was set on fire at regular intervals, burn incidents were not all that commonplace. Many farms maintained a precarious level of fertility by burn-offs in response to the steady encroachment of scrub and gorse. (These farmers were known cynically as 'match farmers'.)

A number of small remote communities were yet to receive the modern blessing of electricity and instead relied on the wood stove for cooking and heat. Candles and kerosene lightened their darkness. At any one time there were a lot of flames about the place, but a healthy respect for fire, learned early, ensured that accidents were fairly rare.

Two burns come to mind. The first occurred a few weeks before I arrived in Kaitaia and even then was gathering the status of a legend. It involved a young man who was sleeping off a celebratory episode in a tent when it caught fire.

Because about sixty percent of his skin was involved in full thickness burns, pain management from hour to hour was a major problem. His shouts and groans regularly echoed throughout the building, alarming the other patients, terrifying the visitors and frustrating the staff. The hospital began to sound like a torture chamber. Normal doses of morphine offered only short term relief. The higher doses needed for more continuous comfort produced profound respiratory depression with the real risk of a fatal pneumonia or death from respiratory failure.

As the level of desperation spiralled upwards, a sudden death in the town offered a possible solution. Bob consulted the relatives of the deceased and readily gained their permission to take skin grafts from the body. Everyone realised that it was very unlikely that the grafts would 'take' but it was well known that once a skin graft covered a burnt area pain was significantly reduced. Everyone's hopes were pinned on this observation.

Great care was taken to sterilise the skin of the cadaver before the grafts were shaved off using a sterile cut-throat razor. These wafers of dermis were carefully spread out on linen coated with sterile Vaseline and immediately applied to the anaesthetised patient.

Everyone waited anxiously for the youth to come around after the procedure. The result was a minor miracle. Only modest doses of morphine were now necessary and a welcome peace returned to the hospital.

The stage was set for the second tragedy in the early evening on a remote farm. It was the 'burn-off' season and some children were having a little bonfire of gorse bushes not far from the house. A four year old girl was watching from her bedroom window as her siblings danced around in the magic flicker of firelight. She could not resist the temptation to join them - and she did so, dressed in a long nightgown.

Alerted by the screaming children, her quick-thinking grandmother rushed down the paddock with a rug under one arm and a twenty five pound bag of flour under the other. She poured the flour over the child smothering the flames and rolled her up in the blanket. By the time they arrived at the hospital the child was remarkably calm. Fluid released from the inevitable blisters had soaked into the flour forming a unique, moulded plastic dressing - pastry.

Today the child would be airlifted to the nearest Burns Unit, but in those days, without any air ambulance services, we had to cope with the situation until the patient was capable of withstanding the long road journey to Middlemore in Auckland.

I rang the experts at Middlemore, but their management advice called for a battery of blood tests to be repeated several times each day. Most of these investigations called for equipment our 'broom cupboard' lab did not possess. Furthermore the child had only a few accessible veins to draw blood from and already two of these were committed to intra-venous drips - blood or plasma in one and electrolyte (salt) solution in the other. As a practical compromise we simply monitored her fluctuating fluid balance according to the specific gravity of her urine - a real 'back to basics' move that worked.

Slowly we struggled to remove the now dry, crisp, pie crust from the body of this incredibly brave wee girl and had her ready to transfer to Auckland a couple of weeks later. The experts there were complimentary about our management - but I put it down to Grandma's flour.

The teams involved in both of these cases had every right to stand on the hospital steps to farewell two people whose lives had been saved - and we were also entitled to a small smile of satisfaction. However, it is too easy to overlook the scars that would for ever disfigure some of their skin and permanently distort the lives into which we had released them.

BOB IS PROMOTED

New Zealand's Far North has many seasons and the weather accounts for only two of them. It rains throughout the winter and a little less often, though heavier, in the summer. Autumn dissolves imperceptibly into winter and spring is a figment of summer. The dairy farmer has a 'dry season' in mid winter when the cows are dry but the countryside is wet. The 'calving season' follows the 'dry season' and the 'burn-off' season follows the 'wet season'. On top of this we have the 'shooting season' which comes in the 'dry season' when it usually rains every day. During the 'shooting season' normally placid, gentle, matter-of-fact men arm themselves with double-barreled shotguns and trudge forth before dawn to blast unsuspecting ducks and pheasants out of the morning sky - but never when they are not airborne. To a dedicated duck-shooter the phrase 'a sitting duck' is one, big, sporting, no-no.

Jo and I were married on the first day of the 'shooting season'. The timing of this event drew the inevitable ribald comments from some of our well wishers, but for me - as one who remembers dates with difficulty - it proved to be perfect timing. As soon as duck decoys and shotguns appear in the windows of sports shops I am forewarned and hence forearmed.

After a couple of years working together, Bob and I began to get on top of a decade or two of accumulated pathology. Bob was one of those rare surgeons who could, when necessary, give a passable anaesthetic and for a time we would alternate roles (sometimes even according to the toss of a coin). Thus I could gain practical experience in basic surgery - particularly with respect to emergency procedures like Caesarian Sections. Also, he was not keen on tonsillectomies and this became my little niche - and remained so for many years.

Before long the local grandparents, uncles and aunts realised that those of their younger relatives who were currently languishing on a waiting list in the big cities could have a quick, free tonsillectomy in Kaitaia. They would invite the kids up for one school holiday and take them to the clinic where a booking would be made in the famous pocket diary for the following school holiday - an arrangement that did not endear us to a number of private consultants in the bigger smokes who had just bought new cars.

As the surgical pressure began to ease, Bob became restless and after a couple of years together my mentor headed south to Whangarei Hospital and well deserved promotion.

His replacement was George Forster, a Kiwi graduate, who had recently completed his Fellowship in General Surgery in the U.K. and now wished to return to New Zealand with his wife Wendy. George was keen to have a job to go to after the financial desert of post graduate study. They landed in Auckland and immediately threaded their way north.

Adrian Webb, our T.B. man in Whangarei, was uncle to George's Wendy and, realising how professionally isolated George would be once he reached Kaitaia, Adrian decided to arrange a 'get to know the specialists', morning tea party for the travelers as they passed through.

From Wendy, George learned that Adrian had been a T.B. patient before he made this disease his specialty. They were the first to arrive and Wendy introduced her husband to her uncle.

The eye specialist was next - Dr. Pullar of the Concord rescue saga. Now, Dr. Pullar wore extremely thick glasses through which he peered attentively at George during the introduction-

"This is Dr. Pullar our Ophthalmologist."

Next up the steps bounced George Wilson the Ear, Nose and Throat man. While vigorously shaking the new surgeon's hand in enthusiastic welcome he was busy adjusting his own hearing aid with the other -

"George, meet George the E.N.T. consultant."

Fred Gruar was next. He had recently injured his ankle in a tennis match and was now struggling into the room propped up on elbow crutches with a leg in plaster.

"Meet Fred our orthopod."

George and Wendy were busy adjusting to this quaint local custom in which consultants reflected their specialty in such a personal way, when the phone rang. After answering it Adrian announced to the assembled company -

"That was our Physician, Clive Garlick - he sends his apologies - he is laid up with the flu."

George turned to Adrian and with all the serious concern he could muster, gently enquired -

"Adrian - please tell me - does Whangarei have a V.D. specialist?"

"Fraid not George."

"Thank God for that."

George adapted quickly to a shambling shanty of a Children's Ward, a broom cupboard for a Laboratory and a two-bed sideroom for an X-ray Department. At least the theatre was adequate for basic cutting, so he could endorse his new qualifications and get on with a bit of surgery.

He was a big, 'huggy bear' of a man, who liked the outdoors. The locals lined up to invite him pig hunting - shooting - fishing and generally made him welcome. We all found the transition from Bob to George a smooth one. The trust that the community had placed in Bob's hands was smoothly transferred to his successor's. For Kaitaia it was business as usual.

Each afternoon at 3 p.m. the Superintendent's tiny office, just inside the hospital's front door, became an informal meeting place between the two hospital doctors and the district's G.Ps. Those with an urge to escape the Consulting Room would call in for a cuppa before setting out on the marathon cross-country journeys that linked up the home visits. Some of the five G.Ps. gave anaesthetics at the hospital, some held regular weekly clinics in the remote corners of the country and all were involved in maternity practice.

On one such afternoon, not long after George had settled in, the boss rang from Whangarei. Rawene Hospital had run out of doctors once again and would I trundle across to fill in for a few weeks until the new appointee arrived in the country?

So I did.

RAWENE REVISITED

The journey south and westward to Rawene was like a homecoming, only this time I was not alone but accompanied by my pregnant wife Jo and our infant Charlotte. Once inside the County Boundary I enthusiastically reclaimed the Hokianga tradition and nodded, waved or tooted to anyone and everyone I passed.

On this occasion we headed straight to the Superintendent's House on the ridge, with its twin magnificent views. There would be no hiatus at the hotel and no disputes over who owes whom a girl and there would be no need for a welcoming committee on the hospital steps - my earlier initiation still held.

Renee, forewarned by her spies in the staffroom, met us at the residence with eyes happily a-flutter in relaxed reunion. Once again I was Hospital Superintendent (temporary), Director of the Special Area (temporary), Port Health Officer (temporary) and temporary Medical Officer to New Zealand Railways.

One of my first official tasks was to attend yet another Hokianga Hospital Committee meeting. These gatherings could usually be fitted comfortably between lunch and an early afternoon tea - with plenty of time for a second cup. However on this occasion there was a problem. A Dairy Company driver, who began his collection circuit in the early hours of each morning, had written a long letter to the committee, righteously claiming to have seen assorted men emerging from the Nurse's Home in the small wee hours on the following occasions. (There followed a detailed list of dates and times compiled with fanatical, perhaps envious precision.)

As this litany of accusation was read out I glanced across the table to Renee and was alarmed to find her cold steel blue eyes ominously stilled by this damning inventory of implied sin. There was big trouble on the horizon and everyone knew it. Ray Cox, who was then chairing about his thousandth meeting, glanced up and instinctively braced himself against the outburst that everyone present now anticipated. The silence that followed the secretary's detailed recital - like the interval between lighting a fuse and the inevitable explosion - froze the meeting in dreaded expectation.

When it came it flooded the room. Everyone mentally grabbed at words as they tumbled about their heads like so much broken crockery - and struggled to piece the situation back into a coherent whole. Renee was very, very angry.

"Who does this sneaky, tell-tale, treacherous idiot think he is? How dare he write such a letter accusing my nurses - how dare this committee receive such unsubstantiated rubbish and allow it to be read out at a meeting - my nurses are far too tired after long hours on duty caring for the sick to ...."

Like a passing short, sharp hail storm, eventually the verbal ricochets subsided. Council for the Defense was at last running out of steam and a very welcome flutter of her eyelids was signaling an armistice. My fellow committee members, once again accurately reading the signs, relaxed back in their chairs and patiently anticipated the tea and scones set out on the varnished, oak, tea trolley nearby.

The storm had passed and Renee's voice was now softened by a wicked reasonableness that gathered acceptance even before the words emerged.

" - and anyway, I will not have my nurses risking pneumonia in the wet grass behind the bushes."

Mr. Cox immediately resolved that the matter be left in the capable hands of our Matron. The welcome clatter of tea cups unanimously confirmed the resolution and closed the meeting.

As we wandered back to the hospital Renee slipped away from the group and headed, with determined tread, towards the Nurse's Home to do a little sorting out. There was no doubt about it, this matter was firmly in the capable hands of our Matron.

THE HOSPITAL PICNIC

Joe Slade, the hospital boiler man, held more licenses than anyone else in the Hokianga County and possibly in the entire country. He held licensed authority to drive cars, busses, trucks and stationary steam engines. He was licensed to skipper passenger launches and fishing boats and also carried on his broad shoulders the responsibilities involved in being the only licensed Harbour Pilot. Joe was even licensed to issue licenses for harbour moorings.

His days were divided between maintaining steam pressure in the hospital's boilers and chugging around the harbour in his big passenger launch (provided he was not needed as a relieving driver for a railway bus or to collect cream cans).

Joe had spent his childhood in the wheel house of his father's launch, learning all he could about the harbour from his dad, who was then the Harbour Pilot and uncrowned king of the Hokianga waterways. Joe - his anointed successor.

During the first fifty years of the last century the Hokianga was abuzz with launches and the district was sustained by regular coastal shipping from Auckland. Very early on in his long reign in the area, even G.M. Smith had a launch built as part of his medical practice. Each year the community held a regatta where up to fifty vessels, decked out in appropriated bunting, would race and generally show off around the Rawene Wharf.

Hokianga launches (like Northland's churches) all seemed to have been built from one plan. They all had long, narrow, easily driven hulls with decks extended out beyond their topsides (reminiscent of the modern aircraft carrier) thus enabling them to carry more cream cans. Their lines also showed generous after-sections to carry cockpit passengers. All of this had to come with shallow draught in keeping with the nature of the waters they plied. By the early nineteen fifties road transport had so eroded the fleet that Joe's boat was one of the few that remained working on the harbour.

Cautiously I floated the idea of chartering Joe's boat for a hospital picnic at Opononi, near the harbour entrance, and immediately secured Renee's support. My secret plan was to time this event for the short overlap between my successor arriving and my inevitable departure, but Renee pointed out that in an emergency such as this we could arrange temporary twelve hour cover through the Medical Officer at Umawera and as director of the Special Area (temporary) my authority was absolute.

So we did.

Fifty or sixty staff and families, laden with picnic paraphernalia, gathered on the wharf under a clear, breathless sky and waited for Joe to welcome us aboard.

The narrow, winding Hokianga is a magic harbour that invites exploration. From minute to minute the intimate view changes as new headlands present themselves, slide past and then fall behind. The ultimate destination remains hidden until the last unfolding moment and every peak and promontory is draped in myth, legend and history.

Throughout the down-harbour journey I was privileged to be in the company of well informed people who eagerly shared the European history of their beloved Hokianga with me. Names climbed out of musty history books and relived their lives as the landscape unfolded, revealing where Judge Manning once lived or where Bishop Pompallier anchored and went ashore to hold his first Mass. The sites of long lost mission stations and bitter battles came into serried focus and dissolved behind us as the countryside slipped by. Slowly the waterway widened and hills, bush-clad to the water's edge, began to give way to pasture and the occasional farm house until Opononi was just ahead and the first leg of the journey drew to a close.

At the wharf the party divided itself into two groups - picnickers and fishers. About a dozen anglers stayed aboard in confident expectation.

Joe approached me.

"Well doc - what do you want - half a dozen big snapper or a dozen or two medium sized?"

Never, before or since, have I heard such an extraordinary offer - and delivered with the casual assurance of a shop keeper who knows his stock well. At first I was tempted to leave the choice with him - but this was too good to let pass.

"How about we begin with the big fellows and then try the for the rest?"

And so it was.

Earlier, while we were approaching Opononi, I had noted a dozen or so smaller craft dotted about the harbour, fishing. Now as we pulled away from the wharf and headed out into the channel some of these began to raise their anchors as though giving up for the day. 'Not a good sign' I observed to myself.

Joe held a deliberate course and we moved out into deeper water. As we approached another group of small fishing boats they to, suddenly began to haul in their anchors as though someone had blown a whistle announcing knock-off-time. We were well out from the shore when I looked back and discovered that we had accumulated a small flotilla of boats riding in our wake and following us in line-astern, like a miniature Spithead Review. Joe was leading his own parade.

Eventually we slowed down, the clutch was slipped and with idling motor we drifted forwards while Joe scanned the landscape with his own version of mental radar. I took up a position alongside the anchor and obediently watched the wheel house for the signal. We were still nudging ahead slowly when the order was given that sent the anchor plunging to the sea floor. There was an inescapable air of precision in the whole undertaking. Our trailing squadron caught up and anchored a discreet distance from us and from each other, like a flock of gulls coming in to roost, obedient to the territorial expectations of others.

As promised, the fishing was good - punctuated by those that got away. In less than an hour we had six big snapper flapping in the fish bin when Joe emerged from the engine room thoughtfully wiping his hands on a piece of cotton waste. With a quick glance he tallied the catch.

"Ok," he said to nobody in particular, "Now for the medium sized fish." He stepped into the wheel house and fired up the motor.

We moved southwards, at right angles to our previous course, with about half the previous flotilla faithfully trailing along behind like a string of ducklings obediently following their mother. Eventually Joe let the revs slip away once again as he pin-pointed his position in relation to the adjacent coastline. A nod from the wheel house once again sent the anchor over the side and our camp followers gathered around in the same respectful formation.

We were due back at the wharf within an hour and, as though anticipating our concern, the biting began immediately. Medium sized snapper accumulated in the bin as though delivered to order. We had about eighteen of these on board when time was up and we headed back to the wharf. As we drew close the shore party was already wending its way alongside the beach to join us.

We were sorting through the catch when I commented on what I considered had been a unique experience. However, I was the only one expressing suprise - apparently one never expects less when Joe is at the wheel. Obviously this man could use his encyclopaedic knowledge to make a fortune by taking out endless fishing parties - but I had the clear impression that Joe would see such excess as prostituting his position and a betrayal of his accumulated wisdom. At heart he was a conservationist in harmony with his forebears and his culture. Under his governance we had taken enough - no less and no more.

While we lay alongside the wharf waiting for the last of the picnic party to join us, I reflected on an event that had focussed world attention on tiny Opononi only a few years earlier. A dolphin that they named 'Opo' had visited the area to play around the wharf and had been encouraged to stay. Most, but not all of the locals were delighted with the antics of this intelligent marine mammal and with the visitors it attracted to their very depressed economy. No one could possibly buy the publicity that this unique visitation generated for the region. Soon, however, the euphoria that shimmered around Opononi became clouded by repeated suggestions that the continued presence of Opo constituted a real threat to the livelihoods of the local fishers who, for generations, had set their nets along the shore to harvest the bountiful schools of mullet and flounder that frequented this part of the harbour. Reports began to surface of gaping holes torn into nets and seas empty of fish. Accusing fingers were pointed at the dolphin and its supporters.

Suddenly it was all over. Opo was dead. Killed, some claimed, by a bullet.

This was the story as I remembered it at the time and my recollections would resurface later.

It was a weary hospital party that struggled aboard and settled in for the ride home. Already the western sky was a-blush and a rising tide carried with it the promise of a quick trip up harbour to Rawene. Joe set the throttle for a brisk pace and we surged up the channel with the setting sun gilding our boiling wake.

It was chilly on deck but I was determined to squeeze the last drop from a wonderful day. With an articulate 'Hokianga nod' I silently requested permission to join Joe in the wheelhouse - ever warmed by the throbbing motor beneath. Joe's nod of assent brought me alongside this remarkable man. After a while he began to share a little of his knowledge of the legends of his ancestors who haunted the landscape unfolding ahead. I was very aware that when a kaumatua like Joe shares such stories, the audience is indeed privileged. These accounts are taonga - as precious as carved greenstone, and must be always be respected and never made commonplace. As the light faded he talked of taniwha and miracles, of battles and rescues.

As others joined us in our warm, hot-oil smelling glass house, Joe fell silent, concentrating now on his navigation. Perhaps, like the fish, enough had been given for the time being. Maybe inappropriate ears had now joined the company or was it simply time to leave the past and concentrate on the lights of Rawene that were now emerging to welcome us home? As the wharf light slid sideways into view I found myself reflecting on Opo and Opononi.

"What happened to Opo?" I asked suddenly, addressing my own reflection in the wheelhouse window.

"We shot it," a calm voice responded from somewhere behind me.

I had no further questions and there were no further answers. Within a few silent minutes we were alongside.

The launch gently bobbed and swayed as grateful figures scrambled up onto the rock-steady wharf and into the night above, clutching empty picnic baskets or burdened with sleeping children. One by one they thanked our skipper and drifted away to light up cars or trudge uphill to home. The picnic was now over. There would be fish for breakfast at the hospital tomorrow.

For a long time I was haunted by that abbreviated wheelhouse conversation and the fate of Opo. It was impossible to escape the calm, matter-of-fact voice that responded to my question with such simple honesty - 'we shot it.' The more I thought about the incident the more I realised that there was something tragically inevitable about a situation that involved a dolphin which had been encouraged to stay in waters where nets were regularly set as the sole support for many families ashore. Dolphins and nets are bad news.

In those days nets were made from tanned cotton line that was strong enough to entrap a school of fish but was no match for the direct impact of mature sharks, stingrays and dolphins. Today's synthetic fibre nets would almost certainly have trapped and drowned Opo.

Nobody could blame a dolphin for being attracted to the flashing prospect of an easy meal already enmeshed in a net and at the same time one could sympathise with folk who found ugly holes in their nets through which their living had fled. These fishers were probably facing bankruptcy through the endeavours of those neighbours who anticipated profit from the same situation. The two ventures were simply incompatible - sadly this was not recognised at the time.

Ironically, the move to have Opo placed under national protection dramatically sealed the dolphin's fate - there was simply too much at stake. Let us hope that we have learned from this sad, emotionally charged incident.

THEIR DAY IN COURT

A variety of Christian religions have taken root in Hokianga. The first seeds were sown by the Anglicans and Methodists. They infiltrated the district by land and struggled to establish themselves up various tributaries of the harbour. Later, Bishop Pompallier, adopting a more direct approach on behalf of the Roman Catholic Church, came in by sea in 1838 and tackled the community at its centre. These confusions of faith eventually settled down with the Catholics claiming the north Hokianga, the Methodists dominating the east leaving the Anglicans to flourish in the south-west.

The Ratana Church was frustrated in its first mission to the Hokianga, by order of Dr. Smith. When Ratana was moving through Northland, having already established a church at Mangamuka, his party approached the rest of the Hokianga via Kawakawa. At that time a number of meningococcal meningitis cases had been reported by Kawakawa Hospital and Smith feared that the approaching convocation could be carrying the disease with them. Legend has it that G.M. sent a message requesting (some say demanding) a postponement of their visit. This was agreed to, leaving the central Hokianga unvisited by the Ratana Church for many years.

However, one religion did manage to unite the Hokianga - rugby football. This sport was worshipped throughout the county with universal dedication and enthusiasm, bonding the district with a passion that was the envy of the assorted clergy.

Now it came to pass that during my tenure, a representative team from the Hokianga was destined to play a rugby match in Auckland and every nurse who was off-duty that weekend journeyed south to support their kinsmen. (In those days a trip to Auckland was the equivalent of today's overseas experience.)

The game was played on the Saturday and the results celebrated that night. Because all licensed premises in New Zealand were obliged to close at six p.m. the sale of alcohol after that time was forbidden by law. This gave rise to a number of enterprising establishments, known as 'sly grog dens', which bravely and illegally ministered to the thirsty populace during the evenings. From time to time these dens would be raided by a frustrated police force who would arrest both the patrons and the management and have them in court to answer charges on the following Monday.

And it came to pass that Renee's entire off-duty nursing staff and most of the rugby team were obliged to delay their return to the more civilised Hokianga and instead appear before Auckland's judiciary.

News of this drama did not reach Renee until early on the Monday morning - just a few hours before the court hearing. She was furious. When I encounted her she was so angry that she had difficulty expressing herself coherently while she organised replacements for her errant nursing staff. I could easily understand her frustration in having to cope, at such short notice, with the sudden absence of about a third of her nursing complement - not to mention the implied shame of arrests and court appearances. With this in mind I offered my heartfelt sympathy and was completely unprepared for her reaction to my touching concern.

"They could have rung earlier." She responded. "They could have rung on Sunday morning - *they left it too late.*"

I realised how much easier the task of re-organising the staff would have been had she been given notice a day earlier - and I said so. Slowly she turned to confront me - her face now crumpled in confused disbelief. In a strangely calm voice she explained, as though to an inattentive child -

"The roster is no problem. Don't you see, they didn't tell me until it was too late - too late for me to get to Auckland in time for the court. I would have told the stupid judge a thing or two - my nurses are good girls - it was those smart Aucklanders who tricked them - my nurses have no business being in their courts - and I would have told him so - but they left it too late - too late and now they have to face it alone."

Her voice trailed away in resigned frustration as she slowly left the room and headed back to her flat where she could grieve for her nurses in private.

As she walked away I had a vision of her in court - hat, gloves, the lot. A character witness for the defense of everyone charged. This lady, who had served in the Spanish Civil War and had coped with the injured in the Auckland Riots, would not flinch from sharing a few home truths with a rusty, old, bewigged judge. Her dramatic view of the situation would have undoubtedly made things worse, but it would have been a day that the court would long remember. The day Renee appeared on behalf of her staff - and told that judge a thing or two.

The embarrassed nurses returned from their adventures in the big smoke on the day the new doctor and his young family arrived to take up the position of G.P. to the town. It was also the day the boss in Whangarei rang to suggest that I consider staying on at the hospital and become permanent in all those roles that I currently held on a temporary basis - and it was the day we declined and prepared to return to Kaitaia.

A CHANGE OF LIFE

George Foster was glad to see me back. He had not enjoyed being in sole charge for weeks on end without time off during my absence. Being the lone doctor in the Hokianga was really a holiday when compared with the same role in Kaitaia. I tactfully did not mention the fishing trip.

Having turned down a future in the Hokianga it was time to do some forward planning, especially after Stephanie, our second daughter, was born. Full time hospital practice had many good points, but income was not one of them. The average waterside worker earned considerably more in a year than either of us did in the hospital providing twenty four medical and surgical cover.

One of the town's G.P.s, Mick Foley, called around to our flat one evening and asked for three good reasons why I should not take over his private practice. Unable to think of one good reason we accepted and I plunged into general practice at the deep end.

Mick had a partner, Felix Montague, who was nearly thirty years my senior. Felix made me welcome.

"All you need is a stethoscope, a syringe with two needles, a prescription for cough mixture and something for the bowels."

But it wasn't that easy. In hospital practice you can play for time - get some more blood tests or another x-ray and look again in the morning. Patients in general practice expect answers and they want them before they drive back into the hinterland to milk a hundred cows.

Those were the days when at least half of the patients in any rural practice had no private transport, so that up to a third of all patients seen on any day would be attended to in their own homes. Country general practice involved a hell of a lot of driving.

Mick loved cars and would have given today's rally drivers a good run for their money - after all he practiced every day. I was about to inherit a regular 'milk run' of chronic elderly patients who were visited by him once a week and were distributed over every part of the district. This extensive circuit of the chronically infirm was to be my first problem.

By way of introduction he took me on a whirlwind tour of the county, hurtling up and down roads I have never before traveled. Throughout this harrowing experience my concern was selfishly focussed on personal survival as the blurred countryside flashed by and impossibly tight corners loomed into view inviting the next all-wheel slide. (Mandatory seat belts were a decade away.) At the completion of the rally I was left with little understanding of where we had been and even less recall of the patients I had met. Privately, I concluded that the milk-run would have to face radical surgery.

A BAPTISM OF SORTS

My first day in general practice began with my first home call. The house in question was only a few miles out of town and I set off with a reasonable idea of its location. Built about the end of the nineteenth century and set back a few hundred metres from the road in the middle of a vast paddock, it was a substantial dwelling that in its time would have been the source of considerable pride. The shelter hedges that once set it off from the surrounding pasture had, after a century of pruning neglect, so dominated the scene that only part of the roof was now exposed to the glance of a passer-by.

The long driveway that linked the highway with the tree-engulfed homestead, was marked at the roadside by a decaying cream stand that had not supported a can in decades. A fence on each side, half lost in cocksfoot grass and wild daisies, bordered what remained of the former tradesman's entrance. The formal, grand entrance of yesteryear, that once swept up to the front of the house and was now overgrown by pasture, could still be identified in parts, like the ghost of a Roman road, bearing testimony to better days.

A narrow pair of wheel tracks, separated by a belt of tall grass, lead to the back of the house and an old wooden shed that now lay like a squashed cardboard box, collapsed down on its contents. The shafts of a gig, saluting the past, protruded into the morning sunshine like upraised arms beseeching rescue.

From the end of the drive a short, narrow footpath, overhung by grass and seed heads, had been beaten into the ground and meandered to the sprawling back hedge. Here it seemed to end abruptly - cut off by a giant grapevine. On closer inspection, a gate of sorts could be identified half hidden by the rampant vine tendrils. With my shoulder I pushed aside the exuberant growth and scraped the gate open. My approach was instantly heralded by a dozen or two panicking white leghorn fowls, scratching and flapping like a scene from a Hitchcock film.

The space between the gate and the back door had once been a small orchard. Now, ancient, gnarled trees with arthritic limbs encased in lichen sleeves, thrust out a few leafy twigs in a despairing attempt at continued fruitfulness. The ground beneath them had been pecked bare of all growth and like a mini mine field was now dotted with the inevitable poultry deposits.

Ducking beneath the convoluted branches of the orchard and carefully picking my way, avoiding the fresher droppings, I reached within a few metres of the back door, when suddenly a magnificent white cockerel, flanked by his two favourite hens, emerged from inside the house to stand defiantly on the doorstep, challenging my further advance. For a moment both parties froze in confrontation. I was the first to move, sending the triple guard squawking into the air in a flurry of attack. Feathers, beaks and claws flashed past my cowered head and crouching body as the airborne trio clumsily hurtled past to rally their fellows.

After a few seconds of immobility I looked up to see a stooped, elderly man, bent like his fruit trees and framed in the doorway. He led me through the bespotted, feather-flecked kitchen into the semi-darkness of a long wide hallway. At the end of it a stained glass front door glowed in cathedral splendor. He indicated a bedroom door and while announcing my presence, pushed it open.

The room was even darker than the hall. It took a few moments for my eyes to adjust and focus on what seemed to be a page out of 'Great Expectations'. A Miss Haversham-like figure lay engulfed in bed clothes and propped up on several grubby, grey pillows. Wide-slattered, wooden venetian blinds stood firmly closed against the light which nontheless escaped into the room through brilliantly intense slits. Bedroom furniture loomed up in the gloom like rocky reefs jutting out from a vague coastline.

With the polite preliminaries completed I advanced to the bedside armed with contrived confidence when one foot struck stern resistance. My sandled foot had impacted with significant force against the brimming, under-bed chamber pot. There was a half second hiatus while the impact wave traversed the over-laden vessel and was reflected back in rebuttal, bringing a sudden, cold cascade slopping over my guilty right foot. With the single mindedness that epitomises courage under fire, the consultation was continued without the slightest hesitation and when my task was completed I squelched, cold footed back into the daylight. Disregarding the orchard minefield and the threatening antics of the poultry, I eventually regained the comfort and privacy of my car - older, wiser and wetter than when I arrived. Baptism was complete.

THE MILK RUN

Radical surgery performed on the milk run that I had inherited from Mick trimmed it back to a radius of about ten kilometres and I was careful not to add any new patients to this weekly routine of 'call and see.'

One elderly couple who remained on the list were Dalmatians. They had emigrated to New Zealand from Dalmatia somewhere in the early 1890's. They were now unable to drive and thus were landlocked in their own home. However, despite the many and varied pathologies that plagued them they maintained a vegetable garden of extraordinary fruitfulness. On each visit, while I examined his wife, he would busy himself filling up the boot of my car with enough garden produce to feed a very large family for a week.

They were a typical 'Dally' couple who had been part of the wave of Dalmatian settlement that began around 1890 and later became a flood that had quickly populated the kauri gum fields of Northland. She, after a life-time tied to the house by domestic responsibilities and thus isolated from the wider community, still spoke English with difficulty - unlike her equally hardworking husband who had always enjoyed day-to-day contact with the language.

Both of them had experienced the pain, injustice and ostracism that befell all Dalmatians in New Zealand during the two World Wars. They and their kinsmen had been wrongly labeled 'Austrians' from the time of their arrival in this country because their home state of Dalmatia was obliged to use Austria for issuing passports - although politically and ethnically they were very different from the citizens of that country. When the First World War erupted in Austria, all Dalmatian settlers fell under suspicion as possible enemy collaborators. A similar cloud of mistrust enveloped them again during the Second World War. Despite the tribulations of the war years, the Dallies retained their dignity and stoically earned the respect of the community. My green-fingered couple, however, carried one deep-seated grudge - they repeatedly expressed an ingrained distrust of the Maori.

I found this embedded bitterness a source of some discomfort and reflected on their attitude as I drove on to the next call on the run - a Maori family of eight children crammed into a small 'Maori Affairs' home. Their father was slowly dying of renal failure and his wife, Molly, performed daily miracles of home management based on their sickness benefit. A heap of vegetables would go down well here.

And so it came about that each week a delightful (albeit a slightly flawed) elderly Dally couple regularly contributed to the well-being of a needy Maori family on the other side of town. Molly never discovered the source of her weekly, garden-fresh bonus and I, each week, secretly enjoyed the gentle irony of the situation.

It was the long buried resin from ancient kauri trees that drew European settlers into Northland and it was the visit of the Austrian warship 'Nivara' in 1858 that eventually drew Dalmatians to these shores. This ship had in its company, sailors from both Dalmatia and Croatia and their reports of prospects in New Zealand greatly interested their countrymen. They had discovered a land where self employment required minimal capital outlay and land was cheap. Word of this spread rapidly along the eastern shore of the Adriatic Sea and the first wave of East European settlers began. The focus of their self employment would be gum digging.

Maori once used kauri gum in flares for illumination, its soot as a tattoo pigment and gathered the fresh exudate from the trees as chewing gum. Captain Cook was the first European to encounter and describe this resin. He found some on a beach in 1769 and presumed that it originated in the sea until his botanists, Banks and Solander, found some jammed in a fork of the mangrove tree and wrongly presumed that it was a product of this plant. This error is commemorated in the name they gave the New Zealand mangrove - Avicenna resinifera - bearer of resin.

Both James Busby and Gilbert Mair sent gum to England and America without establishing a market, but by 1844 it had been shown to be a valuable ingredient in the manufacture of varnish and linoleum and our gum export market was opened.

During the early years, kauri gum for export was gathered from the surface of the land by Maori and sold to local exporters. This supply of surface gum was eventually exhausted around 1860 and European settlers, attracted by the rising price, began digging for kauri gum, using spears to locate it beneath the surface. It was in this way that systematic gum fields were established throughout the Auckland and North Auckland provinces.

These gum fields attracted a second wave of Dalmatian immigrants in the 1890's - just in time for the economic depression of 1894 and a fall in value of kauri gum. The Government blamed the depressed value on over production precipitated by the 'Austrian Influx' and banned them from digging gum on Crown Reserve land - classing them as 'aliens'.

However, to the hardworking, frugal Dally gum digging was not an end in itself. They were more inclined to invest their earnings in land which they would farm when all gum had been extracted. In this way much of the farm land in the Far North came into production and in this way my couple of veteran gardeners had established their farm and eventually passed it on to their children.

SMOTHERED WITH KINDNESS

Forty years ago virtually all accidents that occurred outside the big cities were attended to, in the first instance, by a local G.P. Small town Ambulance Services were manned entirely by volunteers and calls on their time had to be limited to situations where the need for their involvement had been confirmed. It was a compromise that worked quite well in practice when combined with a little common sense. Today para-medics dominate the accident scene. These men and women are far better trained and better equipped than we were and the service provided is more efficient than it ever has been.

Responding to an emergency call was always a tricky business. Often the basic information was vague and incomplete and one had to balance the dangers to self and others, imposed by driving fast on country roads, against the need for prompt attention. At night this would be compounded by never being sure exactly where the accident had occurred. 'A few miles north of the bridge', was often about as clear as it got.

Very late one night a message came through regarding a pedestrian struck by a car on the Ahipara Road - 'just past the quarry". This made it about a fifteen kilometre journey out of town beginning with a good, clear, straight run but ending in a stretch of convoluted roadway. I was weaving through the twisty bits when I came upon a dozen or so cars, parked on either side of the road and a group of about twenty roadside spectators gathered around a humped mass that resembled a small, beached whale.

The night was unusually cold and the gathering - with not one warm garment among them - stood huddled and shivering in a circle around the mound as though it was a campfire. The natural leader of the convocation met me and outlined the situation. Apparently the patient had been standing on the grassy verge engaged in an urgent pee, when a car flashed by and he fell groaning to the ground. His mates had dispatched one of their number to summon me while the others had lain their coats over the trembling victim. Each car that subsequently came upon the scene had stopped to offer assistance, adding further coats to the heap. The donors then joined the spectators who were now committed to a long, cold wait before they could decently reclaim their garments.

I shone my torch on what little of the patient's face was visible between the grass below and the coats above and was immediately shocked by the fixed staring eyes locked in final terror and the blue-black complexion. Surely this guy was dead.

Quickly I began tearing the heap of coats, cardigans and jackets aside - eagerly assisted by their very cold owners, now focussed to reclamation. As the pile contracted and the animated onlookers hastily donned their retrieved garments, the colour slowly crept back into his lips and cheeks and his eyes recovered their focus. He began breathing freely as the last few coats were removed and the miracle was complete.

Within minutes the would-be Samaritans had dressed and departed leaving the patient and his traveling companions with me by the roadside. It transpired that having made their comfort stop and during the subsequent proceedings an oncoming car had shot past , very close to our Lazarus. He had responded with alarm at the proximity of the vehicle and twisted his body away spraining his ankle and falling into the long wet grass. And, as they say, the rest was history.

A STAB IN THE DARK

Some groping about in the dark is inevitable when dealing with roadside accidents at night, however one did not expect such handicaps when making home visits after dark.

The call was to a remote settlement and the house in question lay at the end of a road that was so little used that grass grew along the centre line. I managed to drive to within a hundred or so metres of the home. From there it was a matter of scrambling through high, wet pasture (hopefully avoiding soft, brown, hidden deposits) on a course set towards a dimly lit window afloat in a sea of darkness. Here was a home as yet untouched by the modern miracle of electricity.

My knock was answered by a child holding aloft a lighted candle while peering anxiously into the darkness beyond. He lead me across a gloomy sitting room where the remnants of the evening fire were slowly expiring in the grate. The flickering candle that we followed outlined our forms and sent our exaggerated shadows a-dancing across the walls. He stopped at an open bedroom door and with a silent nod directed me to enter.

The room was barely lit by the orange glow of an ancient hurricane lamp, its light half trapped behind a smoke blackend glass. Several adult shapes sat on the floor, leaning against the walls. One, the patient's mother, labourously rose to greet me and introduced her daughter occupying a bed in the centre of the room. The object of everyone's attention was a teenage Maori girl of ample proportions, disturbed constantly by a rat-a-tat cough.

The examination was a shared affair, willingly assisted and closely supervised by the various family members who emerged from the darkness from time to time. I enlisted the child bearing the candle as chief illuminator as I rummaged through my bag for appropriate instruments and drugs.

The diagnosis of broncho-pneumonia was accepted by consensus and I decided to supplement the antibiotic tablets on offer with an injection of penicillin to ensure some degree of therapeutic compliance. Loading the syringe by jittering candlelight was carefully supervised by everyone present - including the anxious patient. I positioned her on her side - facing the darkness.

A discretely exposed area of her buttock was solemnly prepared with antiseptic and after adjusting the lad with the candle, I placed my left hand flat on the target zone with her skin stretched tightly between extended thumb and index finger.

She glanced over her shoulder just as the candle light glinted on the descending needle and in a moment of panic rolled sideways, significantly altering the trajectory at the critical moment. Before entering her subcataneous tissues the needle traversed the side of my index finger effectively pinning it to her bottom. I had delivered the contents of the syringe before my pain struck.

As I withdrew my transfixed digit - and then the needle - the room erupted in laughter. Their response would have been the envy of any stand-up comic, but it took me a few minutes before I could join in and re-pack my bag with some suggestion of dignity.

The young lady subsequently made a good recovery - slightly ahead of my traumatised finger.

Like most of my colleagues I came from an urban background that had conferred an inbred apprehension whenever confronted by animals larger, or more aggressive than ones-self. Consequently I could empathise with the experience of a fellow G.P., Lloyd Johns, when it came to making home visits that included a walk through paddocks of grazing stock - irrespective of their sex. In the Far North there were a surprising number of homes that lacked direct vehicle access - largely because they also lacked vehicles.

Lloyd had agreed to make a morning visit to such a home and knowing he would have to cross a field occupied by cattle, he made it a condition that an escort be on hand to ensure his safe passage - otherwise no visit.

He arrived on time to find not one but two chaperones waiting attentively at the roadside. One was a pre-school lad of about four and a half and the other his younger sister. Both were clearly excited by their moment of shared responsibility. The wee girl took Lloyd's hand in a reassuring, confident gesture and her brother insisted on carrying his bag. The threesome set off with determined tread through grass so tall it threatened to engulph the youngest member. Casually they threaded their way between grazing cattle, which observed their passing with mellow-eyed, polite curiosity.

When the consultation was completed, his escorts insisted on repeating their protective role, returning a rather embarrassed doctor to his waiting car with all the grown-up dignity they could muster.

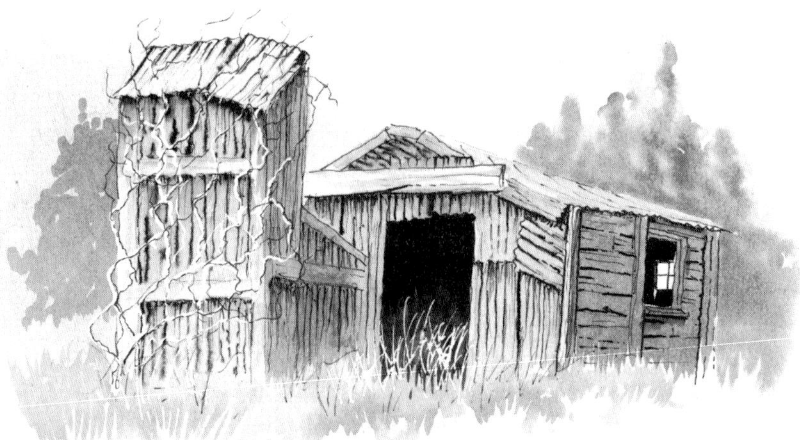

Gum digger's hut Kaitaia.

LAW-AN-ORDER

In the mid Twentieth Century country Police Stations were a law unto themselves and Kaitaia was no exception. The station stood below the hospital on the same hill and occupied the site of the old Redan Hotel.

With foresight that was subsequently forgotten, the founding fathers had prudently built their hotel on Redan Road safely overlooking the river flat along which the business heart of the town would subsequently develop. With typical pioneering ingenuity, based on timber jacks and bullock teams, it was eventually slipped down hill and relocated on the riverbed at the head of the commercial expansion - changing its name to Kaitaia Hotel in the process. It, along with the rest of Commerce Street, was inundated with several feet of water during the very storm that had delayed our voyage north.

The empty hotel site separated the Police Sergeant's house above from the Police Station below and alongside this latter a formidable concrete cell-block had been built to accommodate those citizens who currently faced the law's displeasure. Below the Police Station stood the Court House where justice could be regularly seen to be done - presided over by a visiting magistrate. This layout offered a compact, comprehensive and centralised law and order service for the entire northern extremity of the country.

Citizens sentenced to three months incarceration or less, served their time under the caring supervision of the sergeant and his wife. Escape was not a practical option in a close knit community that could recognise most of its fellow citizens at a distance of one hundred metres. Essentially the Far North is an island bordered on three sides by the sea and guarded to the south by a modest mountain range traversed by only three long narrow winding roads that were easily blockaded.

In the interest of the prisoner's physical and mental health, the vacant hotel site had, over the years, been transformed into a mini market garden through the supervised efforts of a series of shortstay minor law breakers. Each inmate was free to choose between solitary confinement or a horticultural experience, supervised by the sergeant's wife. This apparently attractive outdoor option was marred by the dedicated attention she exercised. She was driven by an unrelenting evangelical force that sought and found constant expression. With a single mind she strove to enlighten the souls of her charges with promises of redemption the moment they changed their wicked ways. It was not surprising that many preferred their own company and declined al fresco Bible studies.

For the district's senior police officer, the setup was the perfect perk. He and his wife rightly received payment for meals and other services they rendered to prisoners - who in turn grew the vegetables on which they all fed. The harvest, excess to requirement, was then disposed of through a variety of channels and the returns dedicated to an appropriate retirement fund.

The criminal mind should never be underestimated and on two occasions, to my knowledge, it triumphed in the face of significant adversity. The first instance involved ten thousand onion plants.

In the last few days of his sentence one enterprising inmate was directed to plant these and began the task under the usual strict matronly supervision. Having established that he was competently fulfilling his chore, his overseer withdrew herself from the afternoon sun and left him to get on with the job - it was after all virtually his last day and she had reluctantly conceded that he was probably beyond redemption this time round.

Now onion plants, after transplanting, lie limp for a day or two until their roots re-establish their function and the plant once more becomes erect.

Each morning the sergeant would survey his neatly spaced crops, anxious for signs of the expected recovery. The first one hundred, planted under an approving eye, obliged by the third morning, but the remaining nine thousand nine hundred remained slumped and exhausted in their rows. By the fourth day they had turned brown, and like their now departed planter were also beyond redemption.

As soon as his supervisor had retired the prisoner had furtively torn the roots away from each plant before carefully inserting it into the soil.

Another prisoner, who loved the outdoors and hated being confined to indoor living, adopted a different strategy from the outset. While freely admitting the evil of his ways he expressed an unwavering determination to make a fresh start, blessed as he was with the promise of forgiveness that such a declaration earned. Whenever he was approached subsequently he reiterated his deeply felt gratitude - by getting in first he pre-empted further evangelising. In no time he found that his porridge came with cream in place of milk and only the finest cuts of meat were appropriate to grace his plate. He quickly became the trustee of the garden.

In his last week he was detailed to plant five bags of seed potatoes and did so with obvious care and skill. He had thoughtfully stacked the bags in the shade at a distant corner and loaded an empty sack with enough potatoes for one row at a time. Solemnly he dragged this bag along each row rhythmically plunging a hand into the bag then pushing it into the raised ridge of soil in the manner of a seasoned potato planter. At each row's end he recharged the bag and repeated the procedure. With his sentence served, their exemplary prisoner was released.

A week passed and it was time for the first dark green shoots to push through and greet the sun - but none appeared. It was well into the second week before an area of soil about two metres square, in a shady corner of the garden, began to rise slightly like a loaf of well leavened bread, raised by the combined energy of five bags of seed potatoes concealed in a shallow grave by a previously unrecognised master of sustained mime.

About this time the practice of prisoners serving minor sentences in country goals was abandoned in favour of a more uniformly depressing punishment (albeit free of evangelic horticulture) in one of the country's larger and less humane institutions. The closure of the cell block as a short term prison coincided neatly with the retirement of the sergeant.

A LITTLE PORANGI

Country doctors have more contact with the police than their urban counterparts and because I did most of the post-mortems I had even more interaction.

Episodes of mental illness cause considerable concern in remote districts that are nearly four hundred kilometres from the nearest mental institution. Once or twice each year we would be called upon to deal with someone who had run off the rails and required management under the old Mental Health Act. On such occasions we worked as a loose-knit team which included the on-duty ambulance driver and mate, the local traffic cop, assorted constables and a doctor armed with enough paraldehyde to sedate an elephant.

Paraldehyde, in those days, was the only medication that worked reasonably quickly via intramuscular injection. It is wicked stuff that not only quickly dissolves plastic syringes, but also leaves the recipient with a painful injection site. It also has a haunting, sickly-sweet smell that is released in the breath and sweat for many hours afterwards. Given the unpredictable conditions that govern such encounters it was prudent to load up several glass syringes beforehand in the reasonable expectation that some could be rendered useless in the struggle that usually characterised these primitive confrontations.

It was very late in the afternoon when the police were first notified of a disturbance in a small remote community. It had been precipitated by the threatening behaviour of a stranger in their midst. He was an enormous fellow, dressed only in a pyjama jacket, and had taken shelter in a derelict house from which he shouted continuous challenges to anyone within hearing.

The team was assembled by sunset and we cautiously made our approach under an unbroken barrage of invective. Pushed into leadership by the power of three stripes, the sergeant lead the way calling out the patient's name with warm (though unconvincing) conviviality. At a respectful distance behind him followed the traffic cop and two constables leaving the rearguard to myself and the ambulance personnel.

The windowless, doorless, shell of a house was spooky in the semi-darkness but the position of our quarry was easily determined by following the flow of insults and threats. These eventually lead us to a room with a single large hole where a window had been. One by one we slipped into the ill lit room and slid furtively along the back wall like the chorus of an opera filing on stage to form a supportive arc around our leader and prima donna. Meanwhile the still voluble star of the show stubbornly held centre stage while backing slowly towards the window space.

A period of stand-off followed in which the uniformed branch stood silently around the walls leaving our lightly-built sergeant facing the enormous, disturbed patient. The tirade eased slightly as its author backed off to sit where the window sill had been, placing himself in imminent danger of falling backwards. Here was our chance. The ambulance driver and I sneaked out of the house and around to the front where the window space was filled by a gigantic, overhanging, bare backside. The rising cadence of voices inside indicated that the fragile trust was once again crumbling. The exposed buttocks began to tremble in sympathy with the ascending level of pent-up emotion. The ambulance driver, with outstretched arms, could just reach the patient's back in a desperate effort to prevent a dangerous outward fall, while I selected a syringe with the clear understanding that this was a one-shot situation. The needle had barely completed its upward trajectory before the medication was urgently pumped home.

As though a switch had been thrown, the mounting level of abuse ceased, but was replaced within seconds by a steady roar as one enormous man launched himself forward into the room, collapsing on top of our trapped and startled sergeant.

Suddenly it was all over - even before the drug could establish its effect. The poor fellow was exhausted and had been running for more than twenty four hours on those reserves of energy that lie beyond our everyday reach.

He slept all the way to Auckland.

Thirty years after this incident I was on a marae in Auckland where I found myself reflecting on this and other similar experiences.

The hui had been called to discuss aspects of Maori health and I was seated alongside a colleague from South Auckland, when a rather agitated Maori fellow began pacing restlessly up and down behind the audience.

At first he simply mumbled to himself as he wandered angrily along his self imposed circuit, but as his courage mounted his observations became louder and more intrusive until he eventually commanded the attention of the entire gathering. The speakers at first struggled to ignore his challenges, but finally they had to concede when the volume and frequency of his outpouring became an incomprehensible flood of abuse and accusation. (At this point I recalled our pyjama jacketed patient and could both taste and smell the paraldehyde.)

Now that the meeting had been hijacked we all focussed anxiously on the protester. I looked over to my companion with an unspoken question that he silently acknowledged - should we intervene in the only way we understood? Sensibly we decided to stay put and watch the evolution of the incident in anonymity.

A Maori woman of mature years drifted towards the interloper adjusting her pace to mirror his. A second woman was approaching from the other side and soon he was being gently stroked on the arms as he continued his verbal broadsides. Slowly his language moderated and eventually he was seated between them allowing his internal storm to abate under the soothing influence of his gentle supporters.

The official speakers quickly regained control of the occasion and proceeded as though nothing had intruded on the proceedings. In the meantime more women gathered around the rogue orator, murmuring their reassurances, reinforced by gentle touching.

I turned to my neighbour and whispered - "We would have buggered that up!" He agreed.

The women sustained their vigil well into the afternoon and were still focussed on their task when the meeting broke up later in the day.

I had forgotten the whole incident by dinner time. After the customary Grace and we had settled down to eat, our once agitated demonstrator calmly climbed into a chair and once again invited our attention - this time to apologise for his earlier behaviour and to sing a waiata to endorse his sincerity and demonstrate his recovery.

I had always suspected there could be another way, but I had to come to a hui on Maori Health to see it so brilliantly demonstrated.

THE HERMIT

The gum digging communities that had been scattered about the North for decades began to experience falling prices in the late 1920's and collapsed completely during the Great Depression of the thirties. Camps of up to a thousand souls, housed in canvas tents and old corrugated iron sheds (and who featured in William Satchel's early New Zealand novel aptly entitled 'The Land of the Lost') began to empty out - only a few stayed on to farm the pock-marked land. Even fewer, with all ambition drained away, remained in the area, sustaining themselves through occasional odd-jobs.

One such fellow was still around in the 1960's. He had continued his lonely existence in a one-roomed shack set well back from the road and surrounded by an ancient, occasionally fruitful, orchard that in turn sheltered a vegetable plot contained within steadily contracting borders. A factor that had locked him into his lifestyle as a hermit was a giant fatty tumour located in the angle between his neck and his right shoulder. This non-malignant accumulation of body fat had grown slowly over the decades until it was bigger than a baby's head, forcing his own head to accept a permanent tilt to the left. This deforming lesion compounded his social withdrawal which by this time was only broken by weekly visits to the local store where some of his old-age pension would be traded for food. Invariably he would be their first customer for the day and back in his lonely cell before other shoppers were up and about.

The week that he failed to fulfill this ritual raised the concern of the storekeeper and after a few more days the police were notified. The grocer's alarm was heightened by recalling that on his last visit he already seemed unwell.

For some reason the police requested that I join the investigating team. Forewarned by previous experience, they had armed themselves with half a dozen cans of insect spray and advised all involved to wear shorts. In single file, our bare-kneed brigade trudged down the long meandering track that linked the shed below, half hidden by the fruit trees, with the road above. We found the door ajar and inside (once one's eyes adjusted to the gloom) a prone figure came into focus, lying in a hammock of sacking suspended from four corner posts securely embedded in the hard, bare, earth floor.

The first footfall to disturb the scene triggered panic in a million fleas. The ground erupted with their sudden confused energy. They rained on our exposed legs like sand particles in a sand storm but their capacity to jump did not extend above knee height. Two constables, armed with a spray can in each hand, kept up an unrelenting barrage of pressure-driven insecticide, while the sergeant and I respectfully approached the bedside.

Near the head of the bed stood an upturned box and on this basic table sat a bowl half filled with what I presumed had once been soup. Its surface was now completely blanketed by a hairy felt of grey mould decorated by a mosaic of other, variously coloured, fungi. This furry repast had been undisturbed for at least a week.

The band of light that fell across his face from the open door was sufficient to indicate subtle, shallow breathing. Furthermore, his head was now centrally placed on his shoulders. The disfiguring tumour had melted away, leaving as proof of its prior existence, a large empty skin flap the size of a dinner plate. His body had been sustained for over a week by metabolising his lipoma in much the same way a camel is supported by the fat in its hump.

In hospital he remained semi-concious. His skin was covered in a fine measles-like rash - flea bites. A significant level of anaemia could be attributed in part to his diet, but his blood had also supported countless generations of fleas. We began treating his pneumonia but after a bed-bath his affronted soul abandoned his newly cleansed body and departed from us and the gum fields for ever.

It was a sad irony that he died so soon after escaping the tumour that had haunted his adult years.

CHANGING THE GUARD

I had barely settled down in general practice when George Forster tended his resignation as Surgeon Superintendent and accepted an appointment further south. His successor was Denis Tree - a gifted surgeon and a fine human being who would serve the district with distinction for the remainder of his life.

Denis was born and educated in England and saw action in the Royal Naval Reserve during the war. In his post graduate years he had worked in orthopaedic and plastic surgical units as well as holding general surgical appointments. He was thus well prepared for his role in Kaitaia.

Moving from urban England to a remote rural district in New Zealand involved significant cultural adaptation but he, his wife Mavis and their two sons, Philip and Alister, adjusted to the strange ways of the North with commendable enthusiasm. Not only did they make Kaitaia truly their home but also successfully encouraged several U.K. friends in the medical and nursing fields to join them in the Antipodes - and in the process enriched the community immeasurably. Eventually Mavis's parents also undertook the journey.

For his first day on the job Denis dressed as was the custom for every professional man in England - dark suit, bowler hat and rolled umbrella. By midday anxious rumour had spread through the town regarding this sartorial assault on our slovenly tradition of shorts and open neck shirts. At lunch that day my fellow diners insisted that it was my role, as his off-duty stand-in, to correct the situation. I argued that because our new surgeon was such an important asset to the district it behoved us to make him comfortable by immediately adopting his standard for ourselves - thus elevating the flagrantly casual dress code of the district to a more professional level. There was predictable resistance to this proposition - even Kaitaia's lawyers reserved their suits exclusively for court appearances and then only when a magistrate was present. Bowler hats were completely beyond the pale.

On the second day of his tenure Denis arrived at the hospital dressed in shorts and a casual shirt and the professionals throughout the Far North heaved a collective sigh of relief. Our new man was adaptable - a characteristic that would become the hallmark of the entire Tree family, endearing them to everyone.

Within a few weeks Denis had been introduced to surf casting on Ninety Mile Beach, had hooked his first snapper and was in turned hooked into regularly fishing his adopted waters. No doubt there were many things that the family missed in their new life but they seemed to find enough in Northland to compensate for most of it. Like all successful immigrants they concentrated on the positive and were soon contributing more than their share to the community that had welcomed them.

While Denis came to terms with the physical shambles of his hospital and began the task of making it ship-shape in the best British naval tradition, I got on with the peculiar dichotomy that was now my professional life - half hospital and half general practice.

I hardly saw my practice partner, Felix Montague, (always referred to as 'Monte' by his associates and 'Doctor Monte' by everyone else). Monte, old enough to be my father, was a gentleman of a previous order. Softly spoken with a hint of English public school, he had a long association with the Colonial Service. His father had been at medical school with Somerset Maugham and there was still an aura of those halcyon days of Empire aglow in Monte. He could swear, when the company was appropriate, but even his cuss-words were enunciated correctly, which, in a peculiar way, made them more poignant. Earlier he had served in various Pacific Islands and probably chose Kaitaia more for its climate than its cultural sophistication. J.T.B. Taaffe (our number one citizen) and Bob Cox the local dentist, were his close friends and this trio made many fishing assaults on Ninety Mile Beach.

One of my first impressions of Monte was his enthusiasm for a proposed whaling station on Great Barrier Island. He urged me to buy into this venture, confident of its potential for profit. (A characteristic of our profession is an innate capacity to financially support off-beat, fly-by-night failures.) I had no problem with his proposition - I had nothing to invest - and of course, the project did fail.

Monte's frank and colourful use of our language managed to give Kaitaia a new phrase, 'D.B. Tonsils', for an old and common syndrome.

It began in Bob Spencer's reign as Superintendent. Monte referred a child to Bob's Outpatient Clinic with a cryptic note:-

"Dear Bob, Thank you for seeing Willie Smith with tonsils like dog's balls. - Monte"

Bob felt it was his duty to inform Monte that the Outpatient Sister opened and read all referral notes in order to organise the clinic. He rang him and explained the situation. Monte was suitably contrite and pleaded that his deepest apologies be conveyed to the staff concerned.

A few weeks later a similar case was referred bearing the following note:

"Dear Bob, Thank you for seeing Johnny Jones with D.B. Tonsils - Monte."

Kaitaia became a world leader in this canine variant of the human tonsil.

In general practice Monte and I passed like ships in the night. He spent his mornings in the rooms while I was at the hospital or making home visits. Things were reversed in the afternoons when Monte attended to his home visits. On one occasion I was surprised to find him still about the place when I arrived after lunch. He seemed to be somewhat concerned - but in a light hearted way.

The first reasonably reliable test for early pregnancy was established in the late fifties - the famous 'frog test'. This welcome innovation was eagerly taken up by the newly emerging private pathological laboratories and cost the anxious patient one guinea. A urine sample was posted to Auckland along with the fee (wet cheques were a recurring issue). The results would be communicated back to the G.P. by telegram.

The problem in small communities like Kaitaia was confidentiality. Everyone employed in the local post office was either related to, or personally acquainted with, everyone else. Furthermore, messages transmitted by telegram were phoned through to the recipient by the local telephone operator and the document involved was posted the next day - small towns lacked a separate telegram delivery system. In this way yet another tier of civil servants were exposed to the information. Pseudonyms, therefore, were essential.

Two days previously Monte had sent off two samples under made-up names and he now had the telegraphed results. One was positive and one negative - but which was which? Monte had been wracking his brains in an unsuccessful attempt to align the names he had made up with their true identity. In the end he notified each patient that their test was equivocal and would be repeated free of charge.

Monte was wiser - and poorer by two guineas.

ONE WHO UNDERTAKES

From time to time every community would need a coffin and when they did they turned to the nearest cabinet maker. Some of these enterprising artisans were prepared to officiate at the funeral as well as provide the burial furniture. Those who offered the all inclusive package deal were said to 'undertake' and were referred to as 'undertakers'. So, you see, it has nothing to do with going under.

The first separation between the two callings developed in urban areas large enough to support a funeral parlour - an innovation that soon became a significant force in the unchurching of death. The transition would not be complete until the 'funeral parlour' became the 'funeral chapel'.

When I first arrived in Kaitaia the cabinet makers who 'undertook' were W. Geard and Son and funerals were conducted either in churches or through tangis on the marae - there being no funeral parlour.

Their business was conducted in their workshop, carpeted with convoluted, fragrant shavings and permeated with an ambience tinged with the hot, sweet smell of horse-hoof glue. The soft light that filtered through cobwebbed, dust-encrusted windows, gave a cathedral-like atmosphere where coffins and kitchen fittings took shape side by side.

The intensity of the father-son relationship was striking. Son Clive was a big fellow, approaching his forties, while Bill, his father, was smaller, frail and approaching retirement. Clive was anxious for the business to explore new avenues while his father clung defensively to the standards and techniques of the past and viewed all innovations as inherently evil. Clive did most of the undertaking while old Bill did most of the criticising.

Their business was both pragmatic and unpretentious. When responding to a call Clive would flick the worst of the day's sawdust from his person, gather up his carpenter's rule, his notebook and the odd form and be on his way - arriving at the house dressed in much the same manner as his grieving customers.

He would adapt his language and bearing to harmonise with that of his clients. Mostly they were either relatives, friends or casual acquaintances. Under these circumstances there was no room for anything but downright honesty. The funeral service would be time enough for dark suits and contrived formality.

Occasionally my attendance at a death overlapped with Clive's initial visit to the family, thus giving me firsthand experience of death as managed by down to earth, country folk. The encounter would go something like this:

"Morning Mary - you'd have thought old George could have waited 'til after Christmas - makes it more difficult for you."

"He always had a mind of his own."

"Any tea in the pot - this could take a while."

"I'll make a fresh brew."

In those days the Maori community in the Far North did not need the comprehensive services of an undertaker. They would simply purchase a coffin and occasionally ask for help with the paper work. I remember when an elderly Maori man died just after his hundredth birthday and his relatives called on Clive for help with the forms.

"What'll we put down under 'occupation'?"

"Hell, great-grandpa had been retired for as long as I've known him."

"Yes, but what did he do before then?"

"Blowed if I know - guess he was a warrior."

"That'll do - *retired warrior.*"

And so it was.

An elderly widow died suddenly in her modest kitchen while preparing breakfast for the only other occupants of the house, her two teenage grandsons. I was still completing my part in the proceedings when Clive arrived. He took one look at the scruffy lads and wrote out two cheques - one payable to the local barber and the other to a clothing store.

"You boys are not going to Nana's tangi looking like that - take this to Cal's and get a haircut and this one to Presswoods and get two new shirts."

To issue a Death Certificate a doctor must have examined the patient *before* death, have diagnosed an illness that could have lead to death and the nature of the eventual death must be consistent with the illness diagnosed. Most of us will die from *natural* causes that have been diagnosed before death. Under those circumstances the doctor will be in a position to issue a Death Certificate and thus avoid the need for a postmortem examination. All deaths due to *unnatural* causes (accident, drowning, gunshot wounds etc.) cannot be issued with a Death Certificate until a postmortem examination has been completed under the direction of the coroner.

A postmortem significantly delays a funeral or tangi, imposing an additional strain on the mourners. The Maori community are especially distressed by this delay and by any interference with the body after death. Coroners and pathologists are at last acknowledging this stress and making a renewed effort to speed things up.

Occasionally the situation can arise where an elderly person, living in a remote area, is dying of natural causes but has not been seen by a doctor for years. Should that person die *before* a physician finally graces the bedside a Death Certificate cannot be issued and the death must proceed to postmortem.

I was on call one weekend when a Maori chap rang from a remote neck of the woods, requesting a visit to his dying grandmother. We both accepted that this was a medico-legal undertaking. Neither the family nor the patient were seeking medication or hospitalisation. The only reason for my intervention was to place myself in a position to issue a Death Certificate when the time came.

The homestead was nearly an hour's drive from Kaitaia. It was a substantial, early colonial building that had been adequately maintained and looked down onto the road and the creek beyond. An ancient orchard, which still struggled to salute each spring with token blossom and a little fruit, guarded its northern face. The roadside opposite was cluttered with a haphazard collection of recently parked cars - many carrying the dust and logos of far away places. All had gathered to share in a death.

The driveway that once linked house and road had long ago succumbed to the triumph of pasture over gravel and now lay hidden beneath the swaying heads of cocksfoot and paspalum. A paddock the size of a football field separated the cars from the homestead. This expanse of knee-high, undulating grass was etched with erratic giant snail tracks of trampled pasture that linked the vehicles with the home - silent evidence of other's journeys. To these I added mine as I high-stepped my way through this sea of seedheads on-course for the front door where a welcoming group was already gathering.

A smattering of adults with kids underfoot, solemnly escorted me to the bedroom that for sometime had been the focus of the gathering. The bed had been pulled into the centre of the room and she lay propped up on an abundance of pillows, facing the door. Like so many elderly Maori she had a dignity about her that we once exclusively associated with royalty. She seemed to be well into her eighties, although her exact age was an official mystery because she had been born before all rural Maori births were routinely registered. She may not have gained a Birth Certificate on entry but we intended to ensure that her passing would be graced by impeccable documentation.

She was dying of congestive heart failure complicated by bronchopneumonia. A previous stroke had kept her housebound for some years. As predicted she declined both medication and hospitalisation. The combined nursing qualifications of the gathered family compared very favourably with those of any hospital ward. Her care was in excellent hands.

Having completed my task I sat on the front steps with the grandson who had requested the visit and we talked about his grandmother.

"You know doc, she had thirteen kids and twelve of them were born in this house."

"Is that a fact - where was the thirteenth born?"

"Under that old oak tree down there - she didn't quite make it to the house."

OF CHAMBER POTS AND ZIPPERS

Accidents, by their very nature, are not funny although an element of humour, on rare occasions, can attach itself to an event.

One night, when on call for the hospital, I received a garbled message about a lacerated, elderly lady who was coming in by ambulance from the North Hokianga. It was then about midnight and the journey could take a couple of hours.

Vague messages delivered in the middle of the night giving advanced warning of events scheduled for some hours in the future do nothing to encourage slumber in the interim. Inevitably, the call announcing the patient's arrival, always comes five minutes after the successful return of sleep.

And so it was on this occasion. At about two a.m. I found myself tucking in my shirt as I stumbled across to the hospital wondering how elderly ladies manage to lacerate themselves in the dead of night.

Half way down the gloomy, sleeping, corridor a slash of light indicated the theatre ante-room where murmuring nurses stood watch over the new arrival. They had transferred her, face down, onto a theatre trolley - a lady of Rubenesque proportions that dangerously overhung the perimeter of the vehicle. The scene was animated with her laughter.

With the easy flow of a well rehearsed performance she introduced me to the rudiments of her predicament - punctuating the narrative with elderly-girlish giggles. It transpired that in the dead of night she had arisen from her bed to attend to matters of personal comfort and had descended a little heavier than usual upon the cold, smooth rim of her ancient, flower encrusted chamber-pot, which, after decades of faithful service, had suddenly collapsed. The impact of its jagged remnant had lacerated a circle in the skin of her buttocks.

The task of suturing this extraordinary wound was greatly complicated for me by her tendency to erupt into deep-seated laughter each time she relived her adventure and shared it with a new and curious staff member. Her chuckles, originating deep within her body, radiated outwards as waves of energy, setting her backside a-tremble like a jelly in an earthquake. This ever-mobile target proved to be a great challenge to my early morning attempts at restorative embroidery.

Gentlemen's trousers underwent occult changes in the mid twentieth century. The button-up fly of yesteryear was slowly replaced by the close-knit teeth of the zipper - a transition that was somewhat slowed by the innate conservatism of the older male. Eventually their freedom to choose was rendered impotent as the button graciously surrendered to the zip.

The early zip fastener was manufactured using brass components and had metallic teeth of significant dimensions. A far cry from today's slicker, finer plastic facsimile. My story involves the earlier bold, brassy model.

They brought him down from the Far North, propped up on pillows spread across the back seat of the car. He lay with his knees bent in desperate search of comfort. As long as he remained still he could cope.

The driver, his anxious son, rushed into the surgery leaving his elderly father, pale and sweating, in the car outside. He begged for (and received) urgent priority and together we returned to the vehicle and its distraught passenger.

More than an hour earlier the old chap had closed his fly with such speed and determination that the brass teeth of the zip had locked onto a small but acutely sensitive segment of his foreskin, leaving a pale fringe protruding from beyond the gleaming brass-toothed grip. As soon as he saw me he began pleading desperately for the merciful release of a general anaesthetic.

"Fer Crisake doc put me out. Please don't touch anything doc, just put me out."

The poor fellow was desperate. Every attempt to further investigate the matter was met by louder and more urgent exhortations for drug induced unconsciousness. In the surgery I had a pair of suture cutters that the manufacturers, in their blurb, insisted could cut wire if need be. This would be their moment of truth. Returning with the instrument I climbed once more into the back of the car where my patient lay, locked in a crouched, defensive attitude, still maintaining his plea for blessed oblivion.

Faithful to the manufacturer's hype the suture cutters easily snipped through the locked brass track at the very bottom of the zip, thus gently releasing the clenched teeth and their grip on his tender anatomy.

A magic, silent moment followed.

The deadly pale tuft of foreskin now blushed with new-found hope and at the same time colour surged back into his face as the brassy prison released its quarry. At this point he would have given me his farm - or at least his new tractor - as gratitude babbled to the surface in the wake of relief.

Reputations may have been based on lesser feats - but I doubt it.

ONE NIGHT WITH VENUS

Sexually transmitted diseases were not a common feature of rural practice and a book could easily be written speculating on the reasons for this. As a sweeping generalisation the incidence would be highest during the last week of December and the first week of January, bound up with the holiday period, the celebration that goes with it and the annual influx of visitors from the big, sophisticated cities further south.

Forty years ago gonorrhoea was the villain. Syphilis had remained very sensitive to penicillin and was practically eliminated, but gonorrhoea was already becoming resistant to this pioneer antibiotic. Large daily doses of penicillin repeated over three days was the currently recommended procedure. However folk who lived in the more remote corners of the district found it difficult to make the required repeated attendances.

A colleague in general practice who had a reputation for pragmatic decisions and the fastest draw in the north when it came to injections, was in the process of treating a young man currently embarrassed by the consequences of his indiscretions. The need for the full course of injections had been emphasised but, never-the-less, he failed to attend for the last jab. This failure was duly noted when the G.P. left the surgery to tour the countryside making his home visits.

Our Romeo was employed in a road maintenance gang of about six workers who were busy clearing drains out in the backblocks when his doctor drove down into the valley where they were working. This was a time in our history when everyone in a small community was rendered instantly recognisable by the car they drove.

The lax keeper of appointments looked up, accurately identified the swiftly approaching vehicle and panicked. Releasing an expletive he dropped his shovel, leapt out of the ditch and dived into a nearby barbed wire fence in a vain attempt to melt into the landscape beyond.

The would-be escapee was entangled to the point of immobility and further struggle simply increased his imprisonment. The car skidded to a stop and the driver emerged from the swirling, overtaking dust, clutching a loaded syringe.

His shocked workmates stood about in frozen postures gripping their shovels and contemplating the evolving scene in silent incredulity. As though in a scene from a silent movie, the doctor, with measured step, approached his desperately entangled quarry.

The needle glinted in the afternoon sun before traversing first into the fabric of his trousers, then the underlying pocket and its contained wage packet and finally the taut skin of entrapped buttock. With the injection completed the entangled recipient fell still as though tranquillised and the doctor silently returned to his car and drove away as though he had merely paused in his journey to gather a few wild flowers.

KAITAIA GOES GLOBAL

The little hospitals of this world rarely interact with the legendary medical institutions of Western civilisation, but Kaitaia did so - and in the process managed to confuse the experts.

Our elective surgical operating list usually began with two or three cases booked in for tonsillectomy which I would attend to under anaesthetics provided by a fellow G.P. When these were completed I would move to the head of the table and administer further anaesthetics while Denis Tree operated.

In theatre we had a wee ritual that linked in with Denis's naval past. When I considered the patient sufficiently unconscious for the operation to commence I would announce "Fire one, Chief!" Denis would turn to the theatre sister and solemnly repeat "Fire one." This would be her signal to hand him the scalpel and we would be in business.

On one occasion the morning's tonsillectomies (which included two classical D.B. cases) had been completed and Denis was tackling the rest of the list which included a young adult with a lump in his foot. The most likely cause of this lesion would be a reaction surrounding a foreign body - the tip of a thorn perhaps - with scar tissue laid about it like a pearl developing in an oyster.

When the operation was completed it was decided to send the whitish, grape-sized lump to the lab in Whangarei for confirmation of our provisional diagnosis.

A week or so later we received a very strange report describing mysterious structures and cell types that made alarming reading. The reporting pathologist concluded that this tissue lay well outside his experience of lumps encountered in feet and was sending it off to Auckland for a second opinion.

The Auckland report was even longer, more convoluted and still inconclusive - greatly expanding the range of possibilities without a commitment to any of them. They decided to enter our mystery tissue into a circuit of pathologists around the world who specialised in the obtuse and mysterious. Meantime the patient had healed up well and was playing rugby. He soon lost interest in the global intellectual storm that part of his anatomy was generating elsewhere.

The hot-shots of American medicine were the most verbose, stretching out the usual four or five line report into whole pages that teemed with intricate description yet only served to widen the possibilities. They were also the first to raise the spectre of tropical diseases and on the strength of this suspicion sent the slides to the London School of Tropical Medicine.

The pathologists who specialised in tropical diseases were just as confused as their colleagues whose expertise centred on cooler climes. Again, strong on description but short on specifics. By and large they took up less space that their American brothers and were more direct in their admission of defeat.

Every two or three weeks a new report from another corner of the globe would arrive at Kaitaia Hospital to be added to the steadily expanding notes of a case that was already cured - but of what? Eventually everyone on this world wide circuit of experts had had their say and the much travelled, much studied slides, were returned to Auckland. They landed on the desk of Dr. Flora Smith, a retired pathologist who had returned to the lab to help out during a temporary staff shortage. Her report, the last one received, consisted simply of a four word sentence which read -

"This is a tonsil."

And I am sure she was right. It is possible that a tonsil removed that day became confused with the lump excised from the foot.

In Flora's day pathologists examined every tonsil removed at operation for evidence of T.B. and in this way they became very familiar with the wide range of appearances that characterise this humble and variable organ. During the last fifty years, with T.B. under much more control, this practice had ceased and a whole generation of pathologists were no longer instantly familiar with the variations encountered in this common organ - particularly if they thought it came from a foot.

BAD BLOOD

In the world of general practice the first appointment for the day will usually be seen on time - with a bit of luck. Thereafter things can deteriorate as emergencies intrude on the vaguely organised rhythm of the Consulting Room and apparently straightforward consultations spontaneously entangle themselves in unexpected complexity. The aptly named Waiting Room soon begins to fill and eventually overflow. Urgency becomes a matter of degree, losing some of its piquancy as the afternoon staggers on.

By mid afternoon the place was already crowded when he stumbled in, fresh from the Airport Bus - and reported to the receptionist. He was only part way through reciting his details at the desk when he began to shake uncontrollably and sag down onto the floor - an episode that gained him unanimous promotion to the head of the queue.

By the time he was seated in front of me he had regained some control over the situation and was able to give an account of his illness. He was on the last leg of a journey home following a tour of duty with the New Zealand Army in Vietnam. On his way through Auckland Airport he had seen the Blood Donor vehicle parked nearby and was so relieved to have completed his service without injury that he decided to acknowledge his safe return by giving a unit of blood. The intermittent attacks of fever had begun later that day and were diagnosed as influenza by a city doctor.

He had reached this point in his story when his eyes glazed over and his body was overwhelmed by an attack of violent shaking. Fortunately as a student I had already seen a case of acute malaria and promptly admitted him to Kaitaia Hospital where the diagnosis was soon confirmed by the laboratory. It was now a matter of some urgency to trace that blood donation before it gave someone a mighty dose of a nasty tropical disease.

It was late afternoon before we had the evidence necessary to notify the Auckland Blood Transfusion Service. Their receptionist was unimpressed by a country quack burbling on about sick soldiers and their perverse determination to give blood. With a reluctance tinged with weariness she finally agreed to pass me on to the technician on duty.

He also had had enough for one day without a last minute call from some idiot in the bush casting doubt on the quality of their precious blood supply. In a bid to shake loose he agreed to pass me on to his supervisor.

My story was well rehearsed by now and flowed with a convincing logic that was bound to command respect. The supervisor listened in silence and then acknowledged the severity of the situation with a four letter expletive and switched the call through to the director.

A rather worried and co-operative director took in the details with commendable speed and set off in a search of the blood unit under suspicion. He rang back half an hour later to say that the blood had been traced, tested and found to be teeming with malaria parasites. He again expressed his gratitude and we agreed that collecting blood near an overseas terminal was probably not such a bright idea after all.

By now the waiting room overflowed onto the front steps and a unit of blood, donated with the best of intentions, had been destroyed.

THE PRESSURE INCREASES

Before he was appointed as Surgeon Superintendent, Denis Tree had gained the impression that Kaitaia was on the verge of having a new hospital built. Such a project was certainly in the early planning stage but a few more years would pass before it became a reality. This delay at least gave Denis the opportunity to take an active part in the building's functional design and thus significantly influence the eventual outcome. With the welcome prospect of a new hospital hovering in the background we, and the community at large, continued to make the best of those inadequate and primitive conditions that still applied.

The post-war boom saw Kaitaia grow steadily. Improved roading began to draw the residents of North Hokianga towards us for business and medical services. As tar seal crept across the countryside small businesses in remote communities fell into decline and eventually collapsed. When a journey to a larger centre could be made in less time and greater comfort than before customers turned away from the local shop with its limited range and dearer stock in favour of buying in larger towns. This mini social and economic revolution left a rash of derelict empty shops and failed small businesses decaying in its wake, and communities that had developed around sea transport became fossilised as road transport eroded their significance.

At the same time and for different reasons, small dairy farms became unprofitable.

These uneconomic units were purchased by more prosperous neighbours to form larger units where economies of scale protected their investment. Farmers displaced in this way found employment in the nearby Aupouri Forest where the twelve week planting season returned more in wages than the farm did over the entire year. It was through this State Forest that social and financial disruption was to some extent buffered within the district, thus retaining a relatively stable population.

Although the district was growing steadily in both resident population and available services, the absolute number of doctors remained static. Each medical practice was steadily becoming overloaded - and, once again, Jo was pregnant, this time with twins.

Monte, my partner, took over her care and in due course she was delivered of Fritha, closely followed by her brother Christopher. All were well and Monte seemed to take the event in his stride betraying no outward sign of stress or concern - but within hours of the delivery he suffered a stroke and was obliged to step down from general practice. Within twenty-four hours my family and my workload had doubled.

The town's G.P.s took turns to provide night time and weekend services at a general practice level. On top of this I was also on call for the hospital every other night and weekend. The stage was now set for a classical case of burnout if I could not attract a partner to replace Monte.

One can wax lyrical about the joys of rural medical practice but the cold fact remained that if the wife or partner of a would-be candidate is not equally sold on the idea, then the prospect is a non-starter and best forgotten. Even finding a locum for a holiday was extraordinarily difficult.

The nightmare continued in a mind-numbing, unbroken routine that alternated between the consulting rooms, the hospital and home to snatch some sleep. The situation was not only stupid but professionally dangerous and yet there seemed to be no escape. Prospective partners enquired, sighed and went elsewhere. The monotonous pattern of 'thank you - but no thank you' seemed to be inescapable until, after two years of trying, I had three committed applicants - Tom Young, Alex Wiseman and his doctor-wife Sheila Wiseman.

Suddenly my cup overflowedand in the delirium that followed I made the snap decision to step down from general practice, handing it over to the three of them and retaining my hospital appointment as our sole future source of income. My accountant turned grey over night.

DISPENSING WITH THE DISPENSARY

The old hospital stored its drugs in an aged army hut - a sort of detached pharmacy known in those days as the 'Hospital Dispensary'. When I arrived in 1958 the place was an interesting and confusing shambles. With the blind enthusiasm associated with the new broom I set out to tidy the place up a bit and sprinkle a few labels on a few shelves.

In the course of this flurry of pharmaceutical domesticity I found many links with a less sophisticated past and one of them was a large, widemouthed jar with an ornate glass stopper. It was empty, but the inside wall was marked with grubby, concentric tide marks that recorded the halting ebb of its former contents. Across the bottom of the receptacle lay several small, discreet dustings of grey powder, each about the size of a sooty postage stamp. A very faded paper label that had already sustained several generations of silverfish could still be read with difficulty. It identified the container as the 'Leech Jar'.

The use of leeches to absorb swelling after several centuries of practice, had faded out during the Second World War and I found this receptacle a haunting reminder of the less romantic practices of my professional predecessors. Indeed the word 'leech', at the time of the Crusades, was respectfully synonymous with 'physician' and 'leechcraft' and 'leechery' referred to the art of healing. (It is interesting to note that in the past few years some plastic surgeons have revived an interest in Hirudo medicinalis, once again employing this blood sucking annelid worm to extract extraneous juices from beneath skin grafts.)

By Denis's time the now cleansed leech jar had found alternative employment and my valiant attempt to impose order in the dispensary had long been abandoned. Inevitably dry rot had taken its toll on the structural integrity of the old building and the continuity of its exterior surface was in many places reliant on a thin, brittle eggshell coat of paint.

The extraordinary success of the pharmaceutical industry in developing drugs that bestowed tranquility had already changed the face of psychiatry and now the general public began to seek access to those agents capable of direct and predictable elevation of mood - and if the side effects included hallucinations so much the better. The young adults of the western world now embarked on a determined crusade to experience the chemical distortions of reality that lay beyond the all too familiar effects of alcohol.

Suddenly every chemist, doctor and vet became the target of violence and theft and before long even hospital dispensaries and the drug cupboards in each ward were included in the new crime wave. The security of all drugs in the community quickly became a serious issue that the police took up with energy and enthusiasm. The old dispensary at Kaitaia that had struggled for decades to keep out the rain was now required to keep thieves out as well.

Northland soon enjoyed the services of its very own Drug Squad based at Whangarei and in due course the sergeant in charge turned his attention to Kaitaia Hospital and the matter of its drug security. With this in mind he arranged to meet Denis Tree and inspect the facilities.

When they met at 8 am at the hospital front entrance Denis was already armed with an impressive bunch of keys that would empower access to all of the hospital's drug storage units. Their first port of call was the aged hospital dispensary. While Denis sought through his collection for the appropriate key the resourceful officer gently took the padlock in one hand and inserted a piece of wire that had begun life as a paper clip. The mechanism obligingly released the hasp and granted them silent entry.

Inside the hut, and securely bolted to its wall, stood the dangerous drug cupboard packed with enough narcotics to relieve the post-battle pain of a decent sized army. Its door was protected against unauthorised intrusion by a tiny brass version of one of Mr. Yale's popular contributions to domestic security. Our resourceful sergeant solemnly slipped one of the then new-fangled credit cards through the crack, released the bolt and silently turned to Denis with a triumphant smile and a well rehearsed, knowing nod. Then, adding insult to injury, he casually pushed his fist through selected sections of the hut's rot-weakened walls releasing shafts of bright sunshine into the building's dark, dank interior. In a voice that echoed the solemnity of the courtroom, he spoke for the first time. - "I rest my case."

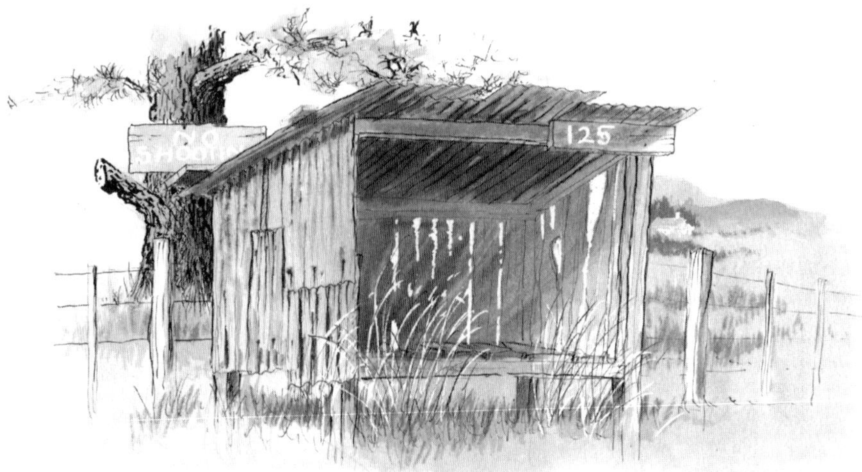

Cream stand.

A HARD DAYS NIGHT

It began with a modest newspaper item that was probably chosen because it was just the right length to fill an awkward space between a couple of advertisements. Had the text been longer or shorter it would not have appeared when it did.

The conveniently proportioned article announced that a luxury, ocean-capable launch had been stolen in Australia and may be headed for New Zealand. This flicker of information, starved of ongoing development, soon faded and died leaving the nation to get on with other things for about a couple of weeks until a cargo ship reported to its owners that their vessel had encountered a launch, miles from nowhere in the South Pacific and in need of diesel fuel. The generous captain had kindly filled their tanks and left them to it. This message promptly renewed police interest in the matter on both sides of the Tasman. They learned by radio from the good Samaritans that the launch they had encountered was similar to the missing vessel although it sported a different name and colour scheme. From the position of the launch at the time of refuelling it was concluded that New Zealand would probably be its next landfall. The police were anxious to establish a blanket embargo on the story while they scoured the coastline for the stolen boat and its wayward crew. Their fear was that should the villains succeed in reaching our shores undetected they could be warned through the media that their presence was suspected.

The remarkable aspect of the story is that journalists and their bosses, representing T.V., radio and print throughout the country, all complied, accepting the police promise that once their quarry was cornered the media would enjoy free access and full co-operation. Today such voluntary restraint would not be forthcoming and not even expected. Times have changed and competition between news agencies is now so intense that it overrides any concept of the greater good.

As it transpired the police had greatly overestimated the navigational skills of the Australian buccaneers. They were next encountered by the freighter Tongariro away to the north of Cape Reinga and wallowing in a state of considerable distress. The fuel they had received earlier had proved to be unsuitable for their motors.

The master of the Tongariro radioed that he had found a launch drifting with two men and a three year old boy aboard. Furthermore one of the men had suffered a knife wound to the upper abdomen and was weak from blood loss. The unhappy trio were taken on board but no attempt was made to salvage the pleasure boat. Instead Tongariro made all speed towards New Zealand and the nearest hospital - Kaitaia.

The operating list that day had already dragged into mid afternoon when the police request came through for a doctor and ambulance to be despatched to Mangonui Wharf ready to relieve the freighter of its unusual burden. As a veteran of the 'Concord incident' a decade earlier I was handed the short straw and hastily began packing drips, plasma, saline and analgesics.

Mangonui Harbour is Lilliputian in scale and comes with all the close attention to detail one expects in a faithful miniature. A narrow road barely manages to squeeze past the sea on the one hand and the steep hillsides on the other. The obligatory hotel, courthouse, police station, professional offices and residences cling precariously to the steep landscape or are wedged defiantly against the bases of the hills. The inevitable general store stands to seaward of the road and extends well beyond the restless tide's edge, held above the wave's grasp by a random series of piles.

Once the home of a considerable Maori population Mangonui has in turn sheltered whalers, lumberjacks and subdividers and yet the shoreline has changed little in one hundred years. The wharf still served an assorted fleet of small fishing boats that continued to gather their modest quota of fish and still return home in time for tea. Mill Bay, tucked just inside the harbour entrance, was at one time packed with kauri logs awaiting transport south and is now cluttered with a range of small pleasure boats tugging restlessly against their moorings.

It was late afternoon when we swept down the narrow road and caught a glimpse of the wharf and the incongruous prospect of a luxury, deep-sea fishing boat chartered by the police from Fullers in the Bay of Islands, tied alongside. The familiar, smelly, fishing boats with their galvanised pipe rails, consistently rusting at every weld, had been crowded aside to make room for the flamboyant visitor.

Motor vehicles packed every parking space along the waterfront creating the nearest thing to a traffic jam that Mangonui had seen since the invention of the horseless carriage. Representatives of the nation's media had arrived in response to the police promise of co-operation in return for the successful news embargo. Journalists and camera crews outnumbered police ten to one. They crawled over the chartered vessel like ants over a discarded lolly. Photographers, armed with their tripods were seeking vantage points around the decks while journalists manoeuvred closer to the key players eagerly anticipating the drama that would soon unfold.

I had naively presumed that our undertaking would be enacted away from the glare of publicity and was totally unprepared for the media feeding frenzy that I had stumbled upon. Any of the small commercial fishing boats that inhabited the port would have been adequate for the recovery exercise - indeed dear old 'Oleo', which featured in my previous escapade, lay to her new moorings only a few miles away. However, the police, in chartering such a big vessel, were honouring their promise and the fourth estate had responded.

As we lay alongside awaiting radio confirmation of the freighter's approach I looked around our floating palace and noted, with some anxiety, the vessel's outrigger poles projecting out from the hull at an angle of about forty five degrees. I recalled Oleo alongside Concord a decade earlier and could imagine these fragile appendages smashing against the vertical steel wall of the rescue ship. With some diffidence I approached the skipper and humbly shared with him my only other experience of ship-to-ship transfers. He gratefully responded to my concern and had these accessories swung inboard out of harm's way.

Radio confirmation of Tongariro's position sent us at last heading out past Mill Bay, through the Mangonui Heads and into the open waters of Doubtless Bay. I noted once again how Karekare Peninsular still looked for all the world like an island as the setting sun and afternoon mist contrived to hide its link with Tokerau Beach - just as it had when we first sailed by all those years ago.

Tongariro stood off, just outside the mandatory three mile limit and we were soon bobbing up and down alongside, dwarfed by the freighter's immense bulk. Cameras clicked and whirred as eager photographers snatched a piece of the action.

A ladder dangled against the vessel's side. I grabbed it and clutching my status symbol, the essential black bag, ascended with an air of casual confidence that was entirely fabricated for the occasion - closely followed by the entire police contingent. The captain greeted us as we emerged over the gunwale and guided me to the cabin occupied by the wounded man, while the police went off to welcome their suspect and the three year old boy.

My patient had been aboard long enough to be freshly shaved and was smartly dressed in donated clothing, which included a tasteful tie. Although pale from blood loss he was able to walk. At this stage his body was still adequately compensating for his injuries and I was anxious to get him away and into hospital before the system collapsed, plunging him into profound shock.

Remembering the circus involved in lowering the patient from Concord and all the attendant hazards that that exercise imposed, I anxiously turned to the skipper for his views on the vital next step. His solution was at once brilliant and sublimely simple. He had already arranged to have a lifeboat prepared for the occasion. We all climbed aboard and the crew casually lowered us into the sea alongside the charter boat. The entire descent was illuminated by more flashes than a presidential handshake. With both boats now riding and falling in unison, it was an easy matter to transfer across and get my patient comfortable. Herein lay a useful lesson that a humble skipper of a freighter could profitably share with the British Navy.

Today we would have had a drip running before we moved him from the freighter, but drip technology was very primitive then, based on ridged bottles and sharp needles that readily broke through vein walls whenever a patient moved. Furthermore, I knew from previous experience that there was insufficient height inside an ambulance to keep a drip running. I therefore chose to monitor his blood pressure and stay prepared to complicate things with a drip if his condition showed any signs of deterioration.

It was during these ministrations that I became aware of the sartorial confusion that my appearance was generating among the assembled company - all of whom were crisply dressed in their best workday suits. I, on the other hand, had come prepared for an escapade at sea and had pulled on a much loved, but steadily disintegrating jersey as a gesture against any risk of exposure during the undertaking. Indeed my dress was so appropriate for the occasion that most of the police and all the journalists had presumed I was a deck hand. My patient, in contrast, could have passed for a G.P. in any Remuera practice. I later learned that some journalists had included a helpful note to their picture editors to avoid any confusion. 'The bloke that looks like a shipwreck survivor', they wrote 'is really the doctor. The bloke that looks like the doctor is actually the patient.'

With a flurry of spray the return trip to the wharf was accomplished in a matter of minutes and the boat load of assorted professionals were soon back in their preferred environment. The whole episode now bore the atmosphere of a completed sunday school picnic.

The journey back to Kaitaia was headed by the ambulance followed closely by the police vehicles. The media, packed into a couple of dozen cars, brought up the rear. Bumper to bumper this strange convoy wound its way through the sleepy countryside like a long black snake decorated at intervals by illuminated scales.

By about 10 p.m. we were back in Kaitaia with two men under appropriate police guard and a three year old boy clutching a teddy bear thoughtfully provided by a sailor on Tongariro. The long night had just begun. The rearguard of journalists were now seeking accommodation and ringing their editors to file individual versions of the night's adventures.

Having handed over the patient to Denis Tree and left the cops to sort out a roster for guard duty, I went home for a quick, belated meal and to get rid of my tatty jersey.

It was past midnight before transfusions and relevant investigations had prepared the way towards exploratory surgery. A step that galvanised the media into action once more. The hospital entrance and darkened corridors were lined with weary newshounds eager for any exclusive crumbs of information they could secure.

By now news of the night's events had escaped beyond our national boundaries and was radiating outwards along international cables. Suddenly the modest hospital telephone system was drowning in a sea of frenzied communication as overseas newspapers and radio stations competed to catch up with the story. A small country hospital found itself at the centre of an information siege.

I gave the anaesthetic and Denis operated. It was a slow business. Each wound had to be carefully explored not only to discover its route and what organs and structures lay in its path, but also to record the angle and direction of the knife's passage. All of this would eventually become crucial evidence in an attempted murder investigation.

The victim's companion insisted that the injuries were suffered accidentally when the patient fell against a knife on the galley table during a storm. The young boy, on the other hand, simply asserted that 'uncle cut daddy with a knife' - but the evidence of a three year old was inadmissible.

Denis was well aware that this operation had both medical and legal ramifications and prudently made careful notes in anticipation of an eventual court appearance. (When the matter finally came to trial he spent three days in the witness box and received the judge's commendation for the clear, careful and thorough qualities of his testament.)

The knife had lacerated the liver and these wounds were the source of the extensive, although slow internal haemorrhage. Neither bowel nor lung had been significantly involved. The prognosis was deemed to be good - and this proved to be that case.

The next day had dawned before we emerged from theatre. Weary journalists, at the conclusion of their vigil, had to be satisfied with 'as well as can be expected.'

Slowly, as the days crept by, these frustrated reporters turned their attention to all aspects of life in the Far North and Kaitaia found itself under a media microscope. One of them came up with the story that apartheid was alive and well in our maternity annex. Another, on discovering a drug company calendar promoting contraceptive pills hanging in the Antenatal Clinic, wrote an erudite essay on the perceived folly of advertising contraception to women already pregnant.

The police wasted little time in charging 'uncle' and arranged accommodation for him in Mt. Eden Prison. The young lad, still clutching the teddy bear, became the star boarder in the Children's Ward awaiting a visit from his grandfather and an eventual journey back overseas to live with him. Meanwhile our recovering patient faced charges of converting an Australian luxury launch to his own use.

The abandoned launch was promptly salvaged by a group of enterprising Kiwi boaties and refitted in Auckland after the police had finished with it. In due course it was delivered back to Australia by a New Zealand crew.

The master of Tongariro was criticised by the owners of the launch for failing to salvage the vessel, either by towing it with them or hoisting it on deck. This was a stupid criticism. They had a wounded man aboard and hours spent preparing cranes and cradles could have cost a life. Any attempt at towing would have called for a great reduction in speed, seriously delaying their arrival at Doubtless Bay. I wrote to the captain assuring him that his decision almost certainly saved the patient's life.

This convoluted tale had one twist left. While the launch was on its way back to Australia, the Australian press picked up the story once again when the vessel was a day or so away from its home port and predicted that an appropriate celebration would be organised by its industrialist owner. With this event prominently forecast in the news an enterprising Aussie rang up a liquor wholesaler to advise them that an order for vast quantities of grog was already on its way and the caller then detailed the quantities to have ready when the company's agent arrived bearing confirmation of the order on company letterhead.

The individual clutching the confirmed order duly arrived with an appropriate vehicle and smartly departed with the booty. Some hours later when the industrialist rang to order supplies for the welcome-home party, he was taken back to learn that a much larger consignment than he had envisioned had already been dispatched - somewhere.

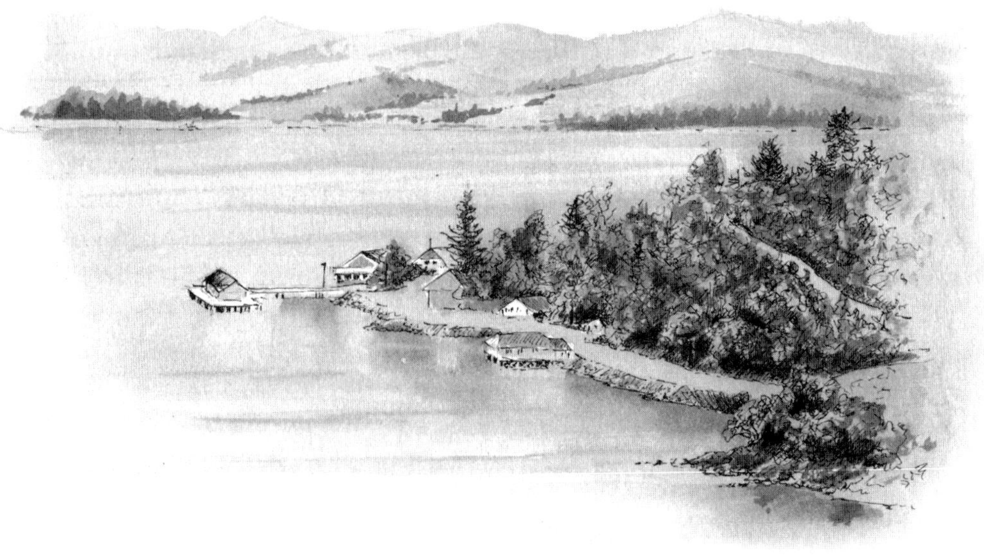

Mangonui Harbour - late sixties.

HIPPIES

Whenever I hear the word 'hippy' I am reminded of a hui held at Te Kao in the late sixties involving ministers of the Crown and local Maori landholders. Discussion had focussed on a strip of Maori land that separated two Crown Reserve blocks at North Cape. The Crown wished to exchange the Maori block for some Crown Reserve land elsewhere and thus consolidate the bisected reserve.

During the course of the meeting many elders addressed the Minister of Lands in Maori and these speeches were quietly translated for the Minister's benefit by a translator sitting alongside. At the conclusion of one oration a rather bemused Minister arose to assure the speaker that if it *really* was the wish of local Maori to have sheep excluded from the area this could be written into the agreement. His response was greeted with incredulity on both sides before the meeting dissolved into confused chatter.

Realising what had happened one of the many bilingual people present rose to enlighten the gathering. He reassured the Minister that sheep would indeed be acceptable, pointing out that the prohibition requested by the elder was directed against *hippies* occupying the land and not against hipi - the Maori word for sheep.

Inspired by the success of Woodstock, high on flower power and hopefully liberated by oral contraception, hippies began moving into Northland in confident expectation of finding their Elysium. James K. Baxter's Jerusalem was their inspiration, the Whole Earth Catalogue their Bible and Hemi their prophet. Northland's abundance of derelict buildings served as an obvious attraction and some small coastal communities did welcome hippies into their midst. Like the curate's egg, they were seen as a mixed blessing. In some places they contributed significantly to their adopted communities - in others they were treated with the smouldering hostility that a conservative society consistently reserves for the unknown.

My first encounter with this new counterculture came late one night. I was driving back to Kaitaia in the rain after a house call when two figures, laden with heavy packs and thumbs extended in desperate expectation, loomed up in my headlights.

Their destination lay beyond Kaitaia. They were heading for a small beach to the south of Ninety Mile Beach. They had no chance of completing their journey in the rain at that time of night and they had not realised that the last few kilometres involved scrambling around the rocky coast, passable only at low tide. So I took them home.

Warm, dry and fed this couple of enthusiastic idealists filled us in with their plans. Their destination was a spot on the coastline where a few tumble-down shacks had once sheltered seaweed gatherers. This isolated area supported a good crop of agar seaweed that had once enjoyed a buoyant market until cheaper imports from S.E. Asia had eroded the picker's returns. Apparently someone had given permission for the group to occupy what remained of the buildings.

To my mind their plans were interesting but impractical - but then I'm the sort of person who looks out anxiously along the wing of an aircraft desperately trying to convince myself that the structure is adequate to keep the plane airborne. Maybe it could work.

Next morning, early enough to catch the tide, we packed them up and drove them to the end of the road, pointed out their route around the rocks and left them like two abandoned kittens. In a moment of weakness we had invited them to visit us later with an account of their progress. It was at this point that we became a surrogate home to a bunch of hippies.

After two or three weeks our visitors returned with a few bronzed associates en route to buy seeds and spades in Kaitaia. Their enthusiasm, fuelled by a run of very pleasant weather, was now at its height. Plans were in place for extensive gardens with self sufficiency the ultimate goal. Minor matters such as nutrient-starved sandy soil, salt spray and steady winds were seen as trifling challenges. Their plans however had one major flaw - everyone must remain free to choose both if and when they contributed their time and labour. There would be no obligation to become involved.

I pointed out that for centuries hundreds of Maori had lived along that coast by arranging their lives in harmony with the tides and seasons, but this was not an acceptable precedent for their community. They intended to succeed without the authority of leadership and if, at low tide, they didn't feel like gathering shellfish, then so be it.

At this stage they were living on personal savings while they struggled to establish their dreams. Although an unemployment benefit did exist it was restricted to a household where the married breadwinner could not get a job. De facto relationships were not recognised. Unmarried aspirants were simply allocated a job elsewhere in the country and given a railway pass to get there. Sickness benefits were likewise restricted to individuals who were supporting the traditional nuclear family. These kids were not in the running for any State support.

Their number fluctuated around a hard core of six or so as disillusioned candidates withdrew to be replaced later by further starry-eyed idealists. Every few weeks we would be visited by members moving south or returning once more with replenished resources and even grimmer determination. The great attraction of our home was the opportunity for a bath or shower and the chance to share in any excess of fruit or vegetables that had come our way. My wife Jo kept a store of tampons for the women. As parents we anxiously observed their self-imposed plight, but in the eyes of our young children they steadily grew to hero status as their clothes and bodies sank into Dickensian poverty. We experienced only one theft and that was a child's toy - uplifted as a comforting icon by a very insecure young lady.

By the time autumn had slipped into winter, bathing in the sea had lost its primordial, romantic charm and each determined survivor gained a pungent aura that was equal parts sweat and tea tree smoke. Extra clothing, tatty and grubby, enwrapped their shrinking forms until they eventually looked like extras in a production of Les Miserables on a bad night. Many took their last ritual shower before heading south on a one way journey.

The few who stayed on were encountering frequent episodes of minor illnesses and a plague of septic lesions as they continued to sail closer to the lee shore of clinical scurvy. They ponged so much that the practice receptionist always gave them the next appointment in the interest of others in the waiting room. Nobody complained about such preferential treatment. My prescription pad plundered the State in support of their languishing experiment by producing a good supply of vitamins for all and extra iron for the women.

Although they had eventually compromised on their stand against leadership, they never wavered in their determination to remain drug free. I admired them for that but the truth was that their pathetic budget could not even extend to tobacco.

Eventually they gained a reputation down the line as a commune where folk, struggling to overcome a drug addiction, could be referred, and a few cases did find their way north bringing with them untold riches in the form of a welfare benefit.

Somehow they struggled through winter and, revelling once again in rising temperatures, began to bathe once more. In one fell swoop they became more socially acceptable and lost their preferential treatment in the waiting room.

Eventually the Kaitaia police began to take an interest in this struggling social experiment, responding to popular rumours that the commune had became involved in drug dealing. As unofficial police surgeon and equally unofficial hippy patron, I was invited to comment. I knew that my reassurances were falling on muffled ears and for a while I heard no more.

Some weeks later a gracious police sergeant conceded with a smile that our hippy friends had been cleared of any suspicion of drug dealing. He had had an undercover cop living uncomfortably in their grubby midst to check out the scene and all he got for his trouble was a dose of scabies.

As 1972 drew to a close and warmer seas washed away winter memories, the political climate also changed. Norman Kirk lead Labour to victory and shook the conventional foundations of the country. Included in this energetic upending of social planning was the concept of the 'Ohu' where designated tracts of Crown Land were to be made available for shared living experiences based loosely on the Israeli kibbutz.

With hope renewed and eyes asparkle, our favourite hippies headed south to transform their commune into an Ohu in Coromandel - and we got back our bathroom.

DELIVER US

It was the first Labour Government in the thirties that introduced free maternity services to all pregnant women in New Zealand. Prior to that policy change fees were charged for maternity services in the same way that they were charged in public hospitals throughout the country. Many families were still paying off debts incurred from the delivery of one child even after the birth of the next infant had added to their financial woes. The Great depression of the 1930's ended with a flurry of building activity that saw new hospitals, maternity units and T.B. shelters erected everywhere - including Kaitaia.

The Kaitaia Maternity Annex stood between the general hospital and the Nurse's Home and remained discretely separate from both. Although administered through the Hospital Board at Whangarei and supervised by the local Hospital Committee, the Annex managed to retain considerable autonomy. The unit functioned as an independent professional body for most of the time, however it did need to defer to the general hospital for anaesthetic services and for the appropriate intervention whenever a pregnancy was not proceeding along normal lines.

This balance between independence and dependence was a tricky path for the sister-in-charge to follow without risking the loss of her basic autonomy on the one hand and ending up off-side with the medical profession on the other. It called for a committed diplomat who was also a competent midwife to maintain the balance. Olive Redfern was such a person - yet another professional, trained in England, who had adopted this country as her home. She taught me all the obstetrics that the medical school had failed to provide.

Olive had a genius for feeding premature infants, inspiring and leading her staff and generating a warm glow of confidence in the heart of every mother who came under her care. This warm radiation was matched by her glorious crown of red hair that cascaded triumphantly from beneath the austere formality of her starched veil.

For as long as anyone could remember the old Maternity Annex had been voluntarily segregated on the basis of its interior allocation of space and the different cultural priorities held by two races. Most of the rooms were single or two-bed units with a rather cramped eight-bed ward at the back of the building. European mothers tended to occupy the smaller units and saw the privacy of a single room as the ultimate in post-natal luxury. Maori mothers, on the other hand, regarded the allocation of a private room as equivalent into a sentence of solitary confinement and resented such placement. They preferred the sociable and supportive atmosphere of the eight-bed ward. The threat of a room 'all to yourself' was bound to secure the co-operation of every Maori mum.

Nobody had ever given second thoughts to this unwritten agreement until the time, refered to earlier, that we had a couple of criminals under police supervision as inpatients in the general hospital and the town was full of journalists allocated to the case.

One newshound, more enterprising than his fellows, decided to investigate the unique ways of the North and found his attention drawn to our time honoured allocation of obstetric inpatient bed space.

His published article decried the Kaitaia Maternity Annex as a classical example of the hated South African apartheid system that was at that time raising deep concern. No doubt some eyebrows were raised further south and a few activists probably took a few notes, but the local response to these revelations began with surprise and ended with collective laughter. Which goes to show how the devil can find work for idle journalists.

At this time the new hospital was being built in carefully orchestrated stages. Eventually it was time to move into the modern, brand new maternity wing and vacate the old annex with its new found reputation for racial segregation. This upmarket unit lacked any suggestion of a communal ward - a feature deeply missed by the new generation of Maori mothers.

The last day that the old wooden annex was occupied was a special day for the Parkes family. All of our children had been born in the cramped shelter of its friendly kauri arms and now Jo, pregnant with our last child brought an era to a close when she gave birth to Deirdre - the very last delivery performed in the old building.

Next day everything and everybody was transferred to the new Obstetric Unit which was promptly blessed by a Maori birth, courtesy of a Maori mum coldly isolated in a single room.

GIVE UNTO CAESAR

Within a couple of years the practice I had handed over to three doctors was down to one. Tom Young was on his own when Alex and Sheila Wiseman moved south. Meantime, as part-time anaesthetist and relieving surgeon I had time to explore, with mixed success, interests such as photography, writing and commercial flower growing.

It was during this partial hiatus that life for all of us was complicated by a family crisis. Jo, who throughout her childhood had been chivvied about 'bad posture' and now, having borne five children, was plagued by constant backache. Denis Tree reviewed her case and discovered that she had a previously undiagnosed congenital spinal abnormality that now threatened to slip and render her paraplegic. He referred her to Ross Nicholson, consultant orthopaedic surgeon at Middlemore Hospital, who concurred with Denis and urged immediate surgery to be followed by nearly a year of immobilisation in a plaster cast from hip to neck. Part of the sentence would be served in Middlemore Hospital and the rest in Kaitaia Hospital. It was a difficult year for us at home and an extraordinary test of endurance for Jo, which she passed with dignity.

With the year of Jo's hospitalisation behind us it was time to reassess our situation. My old practice was now a solo practice once again with Tom Young alone at the wheel. I began to help out with the odd afternoon in the consulting rooms. Tom had brought with him a special interest in obstetrics, paediatrics and anaesthetics - skills that made him uniquely valuable to the district and in time he became an informal and unofficial obstetric advisor to his fellow G.P.s.

It came to pass that one day, not long after maternity services had moved into the flash new obstetric unit, one of the town's G.P.s realised that a particular labour was facing difficulties. He called on Tom for advice and assistance. Tom knew that the next step had to be a trial of obstetric forceps and before these could be applied the patient would need a general anaesthetic and I was called in to pass the necessary gas for the procedure.

However, it was soon clear that this delivery could not proceed safely using forceps - leaving Caesarean Section as the ultimate solution and to do this it was necessary to move everyone, including an anaesthetised patient, up two floors to the general surgical theatre where the staff were already preparing for the operation. Within minutes we had transferred the patient, still attached to the anaesthetic machine, back into a bed and everyone was now crowded around her in the lift.

At this time our new hospital boasted the only passenger lift for a hundred miles and on every visiting hour it attracted the enthusiastic patronage of the district's children. Mr. Otis never had a more popular installation. Because of this hyperactivity the mechanism had begun to show signs of 'over use syndrome'.

With the lift doors finally closed and the obstetric team packed in, the second floor button was confidently engaged. The unit ascended promptly but having reached the second floor the doors refused to open. The journey between the relevant levels was repeated several times, but the system consistently refused to grant entry to the surgical suite. Eventually Sam, our Cheshire born theatre technician and one who was attuned to the idiosyncrasies of various mechanisms, suggested that we descend to the basement - which housed the morgue - and try from there. At this stage I was desperately working out how I could, given the available equipment, perform an emergency Caesar as we bobbed up and down in our vertically mobile trap.

For no logical reason Sam's suggestion was successful and this time the doors opened as though nothing had been amiss and we trundled out anxious to escape before the lift changed its fickle mind and rushed us back to the morgue.

With the patient safely transferred onto the operating table a refreshing sense of relief flowed through me. All I had to do now was to maintain the anaesthetic while Denis Tree performed the necessary surgery. I sat back, adjusted a few knobs and relaxed. However, as we waited in the quiet of the operating theatre we could not hear the usual splish-splash of a surgeon scrubbing up in the outer theatre and Tom went away to seek out the reluctant surgeon. He returned within a few minutes, solemnly sat down beside me and began adjusting the flow meters on my anaesthetic machine.

"Hey, bugger off - I'm giving the dope!"

"You're not you know - we have forgotten that it is D.T.'s afternoon off and he's away up the beach so you'd better start scrubbing."

It was the chief's afternoon off and I did start scrubbing. Happily we ended up with a live babe and a healthy mum - sustained throughout the drama by the relayed teamwork of two anaesthetists.

Having effected the delivery I reflected on the fee I could eventually claim from the State - but it wasn't to be. The original G.P. was due a fee for his attendance and Tom was entitled to an allowance for his opinion and assistance, but I was merely covering for the chief in accordance with my contract and had to settle for everyone's best wishes.

As it turned out this was the last Caesar I was to perform - there were unforeseen changes gathering on the horizon.

FAILED ENDEAVOUR

New Zealand's most northern settlement is Te Hapua to the east of Spirits Bay on the Parengarenga Harbour and, depending on road conditions, a good hour and a half journey from Kaitaia. The school house enjoys excellent views of the harbour, guarded at its entrance by high cliffs to the north and a long, low, silver sandspit of silica sand to the south.

The south-easterly storm that had raged during the night was easing with the dawn when the schoolmaster looked out across the familiar landscape. He was completely unprepared for the addition to the scene. Stranded on the tip of the sandspit and listing heavily lay an Eighteenth Century sailing ship, her bare masts and spars in disordered confusion etched against the sky.

The ship had been named Endeavour II and had originally been built as a film prop in Canada. After filming it had been purchased by a consortium and made to resemble Cook's Endeavour. Some attempt had been made to strengthen the vessel for ocean sailing so that her enterprising, yet unrealistic crew could sail her across the Pacific in time for New Zealand's bicentennial celebrations of Cook's first voyage around our shores in 1769. They planned to put the ship on display at each port visited by the grand old man and capitalise on the unproven willingness of visitors to part with good cash in order to explore a rather tatty replica of her worthy namesake.

They had cleared North cape and under motor were struggling to weather Cape Karekare during the night against rising head winds. Eventually the master realised that he would soon be in a desperate situation if he continued to press on and reluctantly turned to run before the storm. Throughout the rest of the night they struggled to head away from land as the wind perversely drove them shorewards. Before long they had no idea where they were.

Suddenly, just before dawn, they realised that the sea had calmed and was now shallow enough to anchor. Miraculously the storm had deposited them in sheltered waters somewhere along Northland's coast and for the time being at least they were safe.

They rode to anchor, head to wind, as dawn crept along the coastline. As soon as there was sufficient light to illuminate the surrounding landscape they called up marine radio for assistance in identifying their position. Lil Walker in Awanui, just beyond Kaitaia, picked up their call during her regular morning marine radio watch and together with her husband Larry, concluded that the weary crew were describing Parengarenga Harbour.

Indeed they were anchored just inside the harbour entrance having been sucked into this haven during the night by the powerful incoming tide. Relieved they relaxed to their good fortune until the tide turned.

Quickly the ebb tide gathered strength, swinging them around on the anchor and ripping past them with the same strength that had drawn them to safety during the night. The tide was now running against the wind and the previously placid sea was steadily building up steep waves that snatched the vessel against the restraining grip of its anchor. Quickly the anchor warp frayed and parted. The crew had just enough time to report that they were being swept away when the ship stranded on the bar and the radio fell silent. It was at this moment that the teacher raised his blinds and gazed out in disbelief.

Although the hull had been sufficiently strengthened to survive passage across the Pacific, as soon as the vessel grounded, the heavy diesel motor held the keel firmly to the sea floor while the swirling ebb tide tore the rest of the ship away in a stream of fragmented timber.

The message we received in Kaitaia was that the crew had taken to their life rafts in desperate circumstances. We quickly loaded up a county council truck with enough medical supplies to stock a M.A.S.H. unit and hurtled north through the last of the storm.

Fortunately our vehicle was equipped with the then novel R.T. radio and as we lurched and splashed our way north we learned that an enterprising group of locals, driving Landrovers, had set off up the sandspit from Te Kao to the south of the harbour while the falling tide still afforded them a safe driveway on firm wet sand. By the time we reached Te Kao they had made it back with a very wet and cold captain and crew. The only injury was to the captain. He had broken his forearm and now stood proudly with his injured arm cradled in a sling made from the Canadian flag. I couldn't help thinking of Ogden Nash's Walter Mitty - 'only a broken arm - set it myself.'

By further good fortune the ship had grounded in shallow water that became even shallower as the tide receded. Although their ship was disintegrating beneath their feet the sea about them was soon shallow enough for them to wade ashore onto the sandspit where their rescuers found them.

Debris from the wreck was swept away through the heads and then washed back by the surf and deposited along the seaward shore of the sandspit. The masts and spars were eventually salvaged along with some of the rigging and ultimately found a new home on Kelly Tarlton's museum ship at Waitangi.

The flag-decked captain insisted to the gathering flock of journalists that the ship could not as yet be declared abandoned because the ship's pet dog had remained on board and its name had been entered in the ships papers as a crew member. However by this time both the vessel and its temporary canine commander had been swept away.

The strange adventures of Endeavour II had a fittingly strange sequel. The ship's anchor, firmly embedded in the sea floor, had attach to it a very long length of synthetic rope that was buoyant enough to float and thus constitute a danger to shipping. At some stages of the tide this rope could be entangled in the propellor of a passing vessel with serious consequences.

The Northland Harbour Board engaged Larry Walker to survey the waters around the harbour entrance and try to reclaim the anchor and its attached warp. Everyone agreed with the needle and haystack analogy, but an attempt had to be made - particularly as a commercial tug, towing a sand barge, regularly worked these waters transporting glass sand to Auckland. A big damages claim could be hovering in the wings.

Larry was the most respected coastal seaman around Northland at the time. It was the same Larry who, with his wife Lil, had identified the location of Endeavour II in the first place. With provisions for two weeks of patient trawling around the entrance to Parengrenga Harbour, Larry and crew set off from Unahi aboard his powerful launch Oleo - the same Oleo that had once rubbed sides with Concord. Later that day they entered harbour, anchored and took stock of the situation. Larry got out the relevant chart and surveyed the landscape as he recalled the description that Endeavour II had given on that fateful morning. However, once he was in the area he could confirm the enormity of the task ahead. Carefully he evolved a plan for a two week systematic search and identified the area in which he would begin the tedious trawl for the offending hardware and its undulating tentacle of rope.

After a quick meal and a few cross bearings had been marked on the chart they began to raise their anchor. It came away freely enough for about half the depth before it became very heavy. Slowly the warp was worked aboard until the extra load could be identified. Tangled around Oleo's anchor was the bright red warp of Endeavour II's anchor. They had found their needle and were back home the next day.

SEVENTY YEARS AGO

The port of Mangonui, about fifty km east of Kaitaia, was once the 'capital' of the Far North and by 1907 boasted a hospital and a hospital board to administer it. By today's standards these were very primitive times and remained so for several decades.

Quite by accident I stumbled across several volumes of committee minutes covering meetings of the board from the late nineteen twenties to the mid thirties. These abbreviated records, typed on an ataxic typewriter and faithfully pasted into a bound 'minute book', encapsulated interesting glimpses of life in the lead up to the Great Depression of the thirties and the time of my birth.

One recurring problem that frequently challenged the administration involved the matter of canvas repairs. One month would feature the parlous state of the cook's tent while the gardener's tent gained attention in the following month. Presumably the provision of a tent enabled their jobs to be advertised as 'with accommodation.' The debate between repair or replacement could occupy the entire business of the board for that month.

During the period covered by these documents the hospital was apparently lit by acetylene gas lamps. The flammable gas was generated by the reaction between granules of calcium carbide and water. The granules were contained in a lower reservoir and a controlled flow of water drops was released from the container above. The gas thus generated was then conducted to a burner which generated a bright light. Cyclists and motorists for a time lit their way by this system.

A generous doctor who lived in Auckland and owned property in Mangonui, having just installed a new x-ray machine in his practice, offered to gift his old apparatus to the Mangonui Hospital. In order to make use of this modern diagnostic tool they would need to install a generator for electric power giving them the incentive to 'electrify' the institution at the same time. Eventually the board decided to go ahead in the expectation that costs involved could be recouped by charging patients for x-rays at one guinea ($2.10) a shot - which was close to a week's wages for a labourer at the time.

Although this charge was really beyond the means of the average worker many of them did belong to a primitive medical insurance programme. It was common practice for folk living in a particular locality to pay a few pennies each week into a common fund from which medical expenses could be drawn. (The system did not usually cover maternity fees). The various Lodges in larger settlements often offered members a similar insurance package.

The new x-ray charges seemed to work reasonably well but the system ran into difficulties when the authorities tried to charge other hospitals for costs incurred when their patients were injured whilst visiting Mangonui. Apparently the visitors tended to make over generous use of radiology in these circumstances.

The hospital board constantly struggled to collect fees - in particular those for maternity services. The extra mouth to feed that comes as a corollary to this event further impoverished the indebted family. One solution enabled the debt to be reduced by trading firewood, kauri gum and ambergris against outstanding accounts. The minutes often recorded the receipt of a cord of wood. (3.62 cu metres) and the agreed reduction to be credited. For many families it was an ongoing struggle to clear the debt for one delivery before the next pregnancy fell due. This was a time when contraception and family planning were more theoretical than practical.

The business of one meeting was completely devoted to a letter from Colonel Allen Bell - the outspoken entrepreneur of the Far North who coined the much maligned phrase 'the winterless north'. Bell was offering a very generous contribution towards the purchase of a motor car 'for the exclusive use of the nursing staff for off-duty recreation'. The board deliberated on this matter at great length before instructing their secretary to thank the colonel for his generosity and to point out that in the opinion of the board, the nurses lacked the mechanical skills necessary for them to avail themselves of his offer, but they would advertise immediately for 'a horse and sulky suitable for ladies'.

The board's budget, which came mainly from local rates, was significantly enhanced through the proceeds of community fund raising. Before dates were set for any evening event, the organisers referred to tables that predicted the phases of the moon and the time of moonrise and set to ensure that there would be adequate light for the safe return home.

'Basket Socials' for the hospital were popular and profitable occasions. These unique social engagements would be unacceptable today. They required men to pay an admission fee of about one shilling (10 cents). Ladies, on the other hand, were admitted without charge, but were expected to arrive armed with a basket of food that they would share with a partner at suppertime. These consignments of homebaked goodies served as proof of a woman's domestic skills - a sort of carbohydrate equivalent of today's CV. After the Supper Waltz the Master of Ceremonies would climb onto the stage and proceed to auction each basket to the highest male bidder, who would then join the provider for supper and possibly gain approval as escort home.

Soldiers, returned form the First World War had held a 'Smoke Concert' for hospital funds and the proceedings for this cabaret event were accepted gratefully by the board despite the taint of nicotine that came with it. Indeed the board, at one meeting, approved an increase in the weekly tobacco allowance granted to the residents of the Old Men's Home.

In the early thirties, as the shadow of impending world recession spread across New Zealand, the board found that its budget for 'Charitable Aid' was coming under increasing pressure. As the only body in the district expected to respond charitably to individual and family crises, the proceedings of the board became a barometer of relative local poverty.

The system of dispensation was interesting. Approved cases were granted modest sums that were paid, not to the individual directly, but to the applicant's nearest grocery store as 'goods to the value of'. At the same time the local policeman was informed of the grant alerting him to keep an eye on the family and report any evidence of drunkenness or inappropriate expenditure. The concept of the 'deserving poor' was well entrenched and well policed.

The board, facing increasing demands for aid from the community, became aware of the plight of families where the breadwinner was serving a gaol sentence. They realised that these families were suffering more hardship than the incarcerated father who was at least regularly fed and enjoyed adequate shelter.

Deploring this obvious injustice, the board members were moved to appeal to central government on their behalf. Their plea was unsuccessful, so they resolved to set an example of compassionate community concern and resolved to issue each embattled family with free packets of vegetable seeds.

Throughout each year the hospital called tenders for a range of items as diverse as bread, burials for the indigent and anaesthetic services. By comparing the weekly wage of labourers at the time with current rates today it was possible to arrive at a conversion factor that could be used to compare costs in the thirties with those of today. The price of a burial turned out to be very close to today's cost. Bread was marginally dearer and the Hospital Superintendent's salary proved to be comparable with that of a similar post today. (When the x-ray plant was installed the incumbent unsuccessfully applied for a salary increase to compensate for his new duties as both operator of the plant and interpreter of its product.)

The annual invitation for tenders for anaesthetic services regularly failed to attract a competitive response from the local general practitioners. Each year all interested G.P.s religiously returned identical tenders - one guinea per hour. In response the post was simply rotated among them in turn, year by year.

This comfortable arrangement however came unstuck in the early thirties when a doctor, new to the district, had the temerity to offer anaesthetic services for one pound an hour, undercutting his colleague's cartel by a shilling. The minutes calmly recorded this breakthrough in professional fees reduction and without hesitation awarded the contract to Dr. Lange who, I suspect, was destined to play a more noteworthy role later in New Zealand's history.

In 1934 the Mangonui Hospital, together with its Board and staff, was transferred to Kaitaia after a prolonged and bitter battle between the two settlements. The wooden hospital was cut into sections and transported to the new site, but a new nurse's home had to be provided.

This was to be a corrugated iron shed with a door and one window. Some board members were concerned that the provision of only one window was scarcely adequate. After much debate they eventually succeeded in having the contract amended to include a second window. As a gesture of welcome a group of Kaitaia ladies successfully raised enough money to buy the nurses a radio to cheer up their tin shed.

Within one lifetime we have moved from acetylene to florescence and from chloroform to subdurals. Patients have evolved into clients and we have turned full cycle from 'user pays' through state welfare and on to market forces, and in the process police supervised Charitable Aid became the D.P.B. In that time vastly more can be done for the client and vastly more is expected of the hospital and its staff.

How far away now is the ultimate expectation of immortality?

JOINING THE TWENTIETH CENTURY

The slow, steady upgrading of the hospital began in the mid-sixties and seemed to last forever but its implementation did not significantly disrupt the day-to-day functioning of the place - a tribute to the service planning involved.

In carefully orchestrated stages the broom-cupboard laboratory moved into a spacious, purpose-built unit agleam with chromium, glass and stainless steel. This was closely followed by the x-ray department, which gained a state-of-the-art machine on the way.

Thanks to the dramatic effects of the antituberculous drugs, the T.B. shelter could be closed, cleansed and recycled as a children's ward. It took two men with two hammers about two minutes to demolish the rotting nest of army huts that had struggled for years to shelter our sick children. The disintegrating dispensary quickly found a new and secure home inside the old hospital building; a transition that was greatly accelerated after the visit of the Drug Squad.

A new boilerhouse arose where the chooks had once been housed in the old hospital vegetable garden. This tall edifice, with extensively glazed walls looked like a commercial glasshouse standing on end. It proved to be a very efficient sun trap - a feature hardly necessary in a construction built to house coal-fired boilers. It did, however, include the latest in automatic coal feeding systems that rendered the shovel redundant.

Plans for a new laundry complex to replace the late Victorian facilities that had faithfully served the hospital for half a century came unstuck when the Northland Hospital Board realised that at Whangarei they had sufficient laundry capacity to service all other hospitals in Northland. By purchasing a suitable truck they could collect and deliver laundry items to all the satellite hospitals in the province.

This was our first experience of 'restructuring' and predictably it did not go down well. The decision was loudly deplored by every community touched by the policy. A flood of letters-to-the-editor expressed anger and disbelief that an entity like a hospital board could be so lacking in compassion as to deliberately take away jobs from the very people they were meant to serve. We were very naive in those days and failed to recognise the straws in the wind.

The next plan involved the construction of the three storied ferro-concrete ward block that would continue our relentless journey into the Twentieth Century. When this was completed, our working lives would be arranged in vertical order connected by a passenger lift. This lift, more than any other feature of the upgrading, was instantly acknowledged as indisputable proof of the district's ultimate step into the modern world.

Maternity services occupied the ground floor with the medical ward above and surgical on top. The building came complete with a chapel and in the basement a mortuary that even included appropriate refrigeration. By the end of the building spree Denis Tree had his modern operating theatre and the cooks got a flash kitchen. The whole project was completed in 1970.

The shift into the new building was completed with mixed emotions. In general the younger staff loved the new working environment, but older hands missed the comfortable convenience of being on one level. Within the course of each day in the old building one would encounter staff from all other facets of the hospital creating a gentle family atmosphere that was missing when we were stacked on top of each other. However we adapted quickly.

OF TREES AND TOURS

Not only was the hospital catching up with the rest of the world - the town was on the go as well. Dairy farming had been the unchallenged mainstay of the local economy long before the demise of the gum and timber industries. Tar sealed roads were now drawing business from smaller settlements into Kaitaia and the sealing of the Mangamuka route was drawing visitors up from the south.

Phil Quilter, realising the potential of the Far North to attract tourists, began his popular bus tours from Kaitaia to Cape Reinga and back - travelling one leg along Ninety Mile Beach and the other via inland road. This successful venture soon stimulated the growth of motel accommodation and other visitor amenities.

The sand dunes that line Ninety Mile Beach had been drifting eastwards and engulfing farm land for untold decades. In 1922 attempts were begun to stabilise these dunes by planting marram grass followed by limited tree planting. The project became a work scheme during the depression and came to a halt when World War Two erupted.

In 1963 the Forestry Department sent Des Ogle to the district to oversee their new policy of marram stabilisation, followed by sowing lupins and then planing pine trees - thus arresting the sand drift and eventually establishing an enormous local asset, Aupouri Forest. Des served as undisputed king of that forest until he retired in 1982. Five years later the forest was corporatised and sold to the Japanese.

The parallel growth of tourism and forestry brought significant prosperity to the business centre of Kaitaia, but it had little impact on the many settlements to the south of the forest. These communities continued to struggle on at subsistence level. Public Health Nurses, local G.P.s and Maori elders all identified overcrowded, substandard housing as a major factor in poor health statistics and the unsatisfactory educational achievement of their children.

The irony was that we now had a huge exotic forest growing on our doorstep and yet could not build houses. At this time the forest was at the stage that thinning was required to allow selected trees to grow to maturity. These 'pole' trees were mostly tanalised and used as fence posts or kiwifruit supports, but usable timber could be gained from them.

A group of us got together with the express purpose of seeking a solution to the local housing problem using resources that were readily available in the district.

Our voluntary, informal committee included a saw miller, building inspector, carpenter, cabinet maker and a draughtsman. We met for an evening once each week to toss the problem around and slowly evolved a concept of building to a modular design, using wall panels about one and a half metres wide by about two and a half metres high. Each panel was made up of thick battens aligned vertically and edge glued across plywood tongues set into grooves that had been machined into each edge of each batten.

Women who had reared families in remote locations were co-opted to advise the team on layout and their expectations of functional design. I still recall their advice when kitchen bench tops were under discussion. The question was how wide to make the bench; the answer was chorused 'two dinner plates wide'. Bunks were preferred in the children's rooms and space for homework, with a good reading light and desk, was considered essential.

Eventually a set of plans was drawn up so that costing could be compared with that of a standard house of the same size erected by conventional means on a remote site. Our costs proved to be just over half of those for the conventional structure.

Early in our deliberations we realised that the narrow winding roads and dodgy bridges, that gave access to most settlements, ruled out transporting a complete house, but the same unit made up of prefabricated modules and stacked up on a conventional truck could be taken anywhere.

Because our panels were outside New Zealand's standard building specifications, we knew we would need to submit them for an engineering certificate - a cost that was willingly met by the local Maori Affairs Office. A panel was prepared to specification and sent off to be twisted, compressed and generally tortured. It passed, to the great relief of all concerned.

Our scheme, together with the precious engineering certificate and report, was sent off to the Minister's Office in Wellington. Sadly the enthusiasm of the local Office of Maori Affairs was not shared at Head Office. The tone of their ensuing correspondence suggested that they saw us as a dubious bunch intent on exploiting the bad press that Maori housing in the North had attracted at the time and still attracts.

After a long, frustrating wait we received a letter which turned down our scheme on the grounds that although our panels had received an engineering certificate, doubts had been raised that they may be adversely affected by freezing. We got the message.

I was left with the distinct impression that the quality of rural housing was not a priority in Wellington and that any improvement could result in a drift of population back into the remote districts. Instead, job losses in the cities a few years later, precipitated a tendency for family members to return home - further compounding the housing problem.

The same week that we received the 'frozen panel' letter, news came through of a refugee crisis in Cambodia. The Red Cross were looking for medical teams.

So I went - but that's another story.

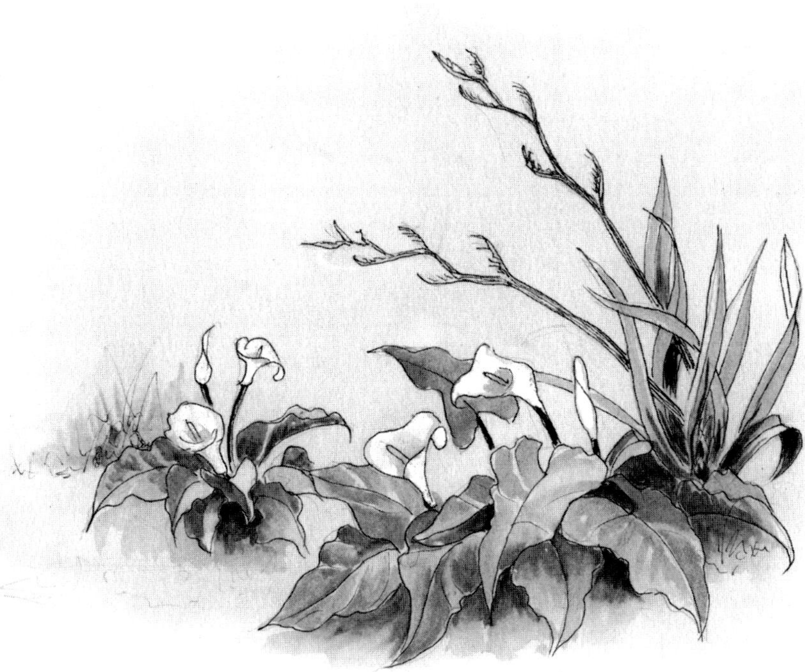